When and How to Use Mental Health Resources

A Guide for
Stephen Ministers,
Stephen Leaders,
and Church Staff

D0018280

KENNETH C. HAUGK, Ph.D.

WHEN AND HOW TO USE MENTAL HEALTH RESOURCES: A GUIDE FOR STEPHEN MINISTERS, STEPHEN LEADERS, AND CHURCH STAFF

Copyright © 2000, 2017 by Stephen Ministries

Stephen Ministries, Permissions Department
2045 Innerbelt Business Center Drive
St. Louis, Missouri 63114-5765

ISBN 978-1-930445-00-0

Library of Congress Catalog Card Number 00-190102
Printed in the United States of America.

17
05

To Stephen Leaders
whose tireless efforts give birth
to Stephen Ministry in their congregations

To Stephen Ministers
who give of themselves selflessly
to bring Christ's care to those in need

To care receivers
(and I've learned over the years that all
of us are care receivers at one time or another)
whose courage in the face of adversity bears
witness to Jesus' healing power still active in our world

This book is dedicated.

Contents

Acknowledgments

This book has been very much a team effort. From the time I first had the idea for this book until the day of its publication, many gifted people have had a hand in researching, writing, editing, and proofreading. I especially acknowledge and thank Scott Perry, William McKay, Vern Koehlinger, David Paap, Michael Welch, Wanda Stahl, and Sandy Ashby for their significant contributions to this work.

I am grateful to the many mental health professionals—clinical psychologists, clinical social workers, counselors, marriage and family counselors, and psychiatrists—who reviewed this book and gave very helpful feedback.

The entire staff at Stephen Ministries St. Louis, particularly my assistants Jeanette Rudder, Lori Kem, Liz Schaus, and John Kahler, have provided encouragement, ideas, help, and koinonia in Christ in a thousand different ways. I consider myself privileged to work with them and I thank them.

Finally, my family—Joan, Charity, and Amity—provides an unending source of love and support. I am especially grateful to them.

Introduction

Stephen Ministry is distinctively Christian caregiving for people going through difficult times or who are otherwise in need of support in their lives. A Stephen Minister often comes alongside a person whose life has been turned topsy-turvy by a crisis or tragedy and cares for that person as he or she puts his or her life back together.

Sometimes, however, a person's troubles push him or her beyond where a Stephen Minister can help. When that happens, the person needs the care of a mental health professional. The determining factor is the person's internal reaction to the crisis—how difficult the crisis is for him or her to deal with. One person might be able to handle a crisis that would completely overwhelm another person. When a crisis pushes a person beyond his or her ability to cope, that person needs a mental health professional's care.

The purpose of this book is to help Stephen Ministers, Stephen Leaders, Referrals Coordinators, Supervision Group Facilitators, and members of church staffs know when and how to involve mental health professionals in caregiving situations.

The terminology in this purpose statement is familiar to Stephen Ministers and Stephen Leaders—the main audience of this book—but there are readers who will not know the terms. For them, here are some definitions.

- **Stephen Series.** The Stephen Series is a complete system of training and organizing lay persons to offer caregiving ministry in and around their congregations.

- **Stephen Ministers.** Stephen Ministers are lay caregivers trained by Stephen Leaders in their congregation or organization. They make an initial two-year commitment to training and service, and very often serve beyond two years. After their first 50 hours of training, they begin caring for a care receiver and participate in twice-monthly peer supervision and continuing education.

- **Stephen Leaders.** Stephen Leaders are chosen by their congregations to implement and manage Stephen Ministry. Stephen Ministries St. Louis trains them at Leader's Training Courses in how to recruit, select, train, and supervise Stephen Ministers. Stephen Leaders are supervised by their local congregation or by their other officially enrolled ministry organization.

To Mental Health Professionals

Stephen Ministries was founded in 1975 by the Rev. Kenneth C. Haugk, Ph.D., a pastor and clinical psychologist. This is a Christian, not-for-profit training and educational ministry organization based in St. Louis. Stephen Ministries St. Louis trains church staff and lay leaders to implement caring ministries in their congregations or other organizations that enroll in the Stephen Series.

Those referred for care in Stephen Ministry are called care receivers. These are people facing difficult life experiences who need a listening ear, a shoulder to lean on, and another set of hands lifted in prayer. Care receivers accurately perceive reality and their basic coping skills are intact. They can control their responses to their difficult emotions and meet their daily responsibilities. Even without the care of a Stephen Minister, they would probably be able to make it through their difficult times, but the Stephen Minister helps carry their burdens

- **Referrals Coordinator.** In a congregation with Stephen Ministry, the Referrals Coordinator matches potential care

  | and assists them in finding spiritual and personal wholeness and growth. |

  receivers with available Stephen Ministers. The Referrals Coordinator is a Stephen Leader who makes certain that a possible referral is appropriate.

- **Supervision Group Facilitator.** Stephen Ministers meet for peer supervision twice a month in small groups of five to seven. A Supervision Group Facilitator leads each group. Supervision Group Facilitators are either Stephen Leaders or Stephen Ministers who have received extra training for this role.

- **Mental health professionals.** Mental health professionals include clinical psychologists, marriage and family counselors, pastoral counselors, psychiatric nurses, psychiatrists, social workers, and other professional caregivers.

Who Should Read This Book?

Stephen Ministers are the primary readership for *When and How to Use Mental Health Resources,* and the references to "you" beginning in chapter 1 can always be taken to mean Stephen Ministers. Stephen Ministers are quite naturally eager to cause no harm in their caregiving. They do not want to get involved in caregiving that is beyond their training and capabilities, and this book erects several safeguards to help them avoid that.

There are others who will benefit from the content of this book, and it is for them as well.

- **Stephen Leaders.** Since it is highly probable that mental health issues—various needs for consultation or caregiving from mental health professionals—will occasionally surface in the course of Stephen Ministry, this book is

---

essential for Stephen Leaders. When a care receiver's reaction to a particular situation becomes more than he or she can handle, or when a care receiver's struggles are much deeper than were originally thought, this reference book will guide Stephen Leaders to take the correct actions.

- **Pastors and other church staff.** Pastors and other staff members are vital to a congregation's Stephen Ministry, even if they are not Stephen Leaders. This book will raise their confidence, assuring them that Stephen Ministry will not go beyond its clear purpose. It will equip pastors and church staff to guide and consult when questions arise about what kind of care is appropriate.

- **Key lay leaders.** Lay leaders also must have confidence that Stephen Ministry knows its limitations in order for them to give their full support to a congregation's Stephen Ministry. Their support can influence whether the congregation will accept Stephen Ministry and embrace it for those needing care.

To Pastors and Other Church Staff, Key Lay Leaders, and Mental Health Professionals

Stephen Ministry training topics include:

- The person of the caregiver
- Dealing with feelings
- Listening
- Distinctively Christian caregiving
- Process-oriented caregiving
- Christian assertiveness
- Maintaining boundaries
- Crisis theory and practice
- Maintaining confidentiality
- Telecare
- Using mental health professionals and other community resources
- Ministering to grieving persons
- Helping those experiencing depression receive appropriate care
- Helping suicidal persons get the help they need
- Bringing closure to a caring relationship
- Participating in supervision
- How to make a first caring visit

• **Mental health professionals.** By reading this book, mental health professionals can gain a fuller understanding of the type of caregiving that happens in Stephen Ministry. They also learn how Stephen Ministry at times can complement and enhance a caregiving regimen they have established with a client. In addition, mental health professionals will better understand how they can assist congregations by being available for consultations, continuing education, and referrals.

• Following Jesus in caregiving
• Ministering to the dying, their family, and friends
• Caring for people before, during, and after hospitalization
• Ministering to those experiencing losses related to aging
• Ministering to those needing long-term care
• Ministering to those experiencing separation and divorce
• Caring when childbirth turns into a crisis
• Providing spiritual care

All these just named are reading this book over the shoulder of the Stephen Ministers, as it were. From time to time, there will be particular messages for one or another of these other readers, in which case they will be addressed from within a sidebar, like the one on these two pages.

Mental health practices and the availability of services differ in each state and country. No matter where a congregation is located, however, the suggestions in this book can help it find qualified mental health professionals and establish relationships with them. *When and How to Use Mental Health Resources* helps congregations answer challenging questions and make the best mental health referrals possible.

How to Use the Appendices

Congregations enrolled in the Stephen Series may adapt and reproduce the five appendices of this book.

- "Focus Question Set H: Focus on a Possible Mental Health Referral" (Appendix A)
- "Confidential Stephen Ministry Mental Health Referral Record" (Appendix B)
- "Sample Letter to a Mental Health Professional" (Appendix C)
- "Mental Health Resource Information Form" (Appendix D)
- "Agreement to Receive Care" (Appendix E)

These documents help Stephen Leaders manage and administer Stephen Ministry and help them communicate with mental health professionals.

Ways Mental Health Professionals Can Help Stephen Ministry

There are three basic ways mental health professionals can be of help to Stephen Ministry—for consultation, referral, and continuing education.

Consultation Regarding a Particular Care Receiver

Pastors, other church staff, and Stephen Leaders can receive consultation from a mental health professional to determine the right care for a particular care receiver in several circumstances.

- After a preparation interview of a possible care receiver, if the Referrals Coordinator is unsure about the appropriateness of Stephen Ministry for the care receiver
- During a Stephen Ministry relationship, when a Stephen

Minister believes that a care receiver needs more than he or she can provide

• When a new series of crises sends a care receiver who had been coping fairly well into a tailspin

Referring a Care Receiver to a Mental Health Professional

A mental health professional's input is very important when it's necessary to refer a care receiver for professional care. Chapters 2, 5, and 6 have more to say about how to involve mental health professionals in such referrals.

Training and Continuing Education

The third way mental health professionals can be useful is for training and continuing education. Stephen Leaders may invite mental health professionals to speak at Stephen Ministry training or continuing education sessions, or Stephen Ministers may suggest this because of particular needs appearing in their caring relationship. If several Stephen Ministers have raised questions on a particular subject during peer supervision (for example, serious emotional disturbances, signs of substance abuse, family violence or other specific family issues), the Stephen Leader who serves as

To the Stephen Leader

There are several key points to remember when planning for a continuing education presentation by a mental health professional. He or she must be:

• clear about the place and function of Stephen Ministry among caregiving options;

• respectful of the perspective of Stephen Ministry and your congregation's beliefs;

• sure that the training presentation is suitable for an audience of lay caregivers; and

• well-informed about any compensation for the presentation, and whether it is

Continuing Education Coordinator could then seek out a mental health professional to speak to the group on that particular topic.

appropriate to distribute literature promoting his or her practice.

• • •

Equipped with the knowledge and resources outlined in this book, Stephen Ministry congregations will be better informed about the various types of professional care available to those the congregation serves and about how to access that care. They can help care receivers choose care that best meets their needs and most effectively promotes their return to wholeness. Equipped with this knowledge, congregations can avoid unwise or untimely assignments to Stephen Ministers that add unnecessary stress to their caring ministry and result in people's not receiving the best care possible for their situations.

1

Who Are Stephen Ministers?

Stephen Ministers are lay Christians carefully recruited, selected, trained, commissioned, and supervised for lay caring ministry.

A Closer Look at Stephen Ministers

Here is more information about parts of that definition.

Lay Caregivers

Stephen Ministers are lay caregivers, not pastors or clinical specialists. They may work as hairdressers or lawyers, bankers or teachers, homemakers, construction workers, or salespersons. In addition to their occupation, they volunteer as lay caregivers in congregations and organizations enrolled in the Stephen Series.

The fact that Stephen Ministers are volunteer lay caregivers is good news for congregations. The cost of employing professional caregivers, both clergy and others, is high, and it continues to increase. There will never be enough professional caregivers available to handle the caregiving needs in congregations and communities. Fortunately many people who need care do not require professional caregivers. Stephen Ministers are qualified and able to meet the needs of a large majority of those who need care, and they are trained to recognize when they are over their heads.

As lay caregivers, Stephen Ministers never accept payment, barter, or any other form of remuneration for their services. To do so would be completely contrary to Stephen Ministry and might damage caring relationships.

Christian Caregivers

Stephen Ministers are Christian caregivers. If the lay status of Stephen Ministers is good news for congregations, their Christian status is great news for the world.

God has so designed the church that all its members have a part in one or more servant ministries, including those involved with caregiving. As the Bible states, "We have different gifts, according to the grace given us" (Romans 12:6a). The spiritual gifts of Stephen Ministers prepare them for, and point them toward, caring for the suffering, the same ministry that Jesus proclaimed as his when he read from the prophet Isaiah in the synagogue in Nazareth:

"The Spirit of the Lord is upon me,
　because he has anointed me
　　to bring good news to the poor.
He has sent me to proclaim release to the captives
　and recovery of sight to the blind,
　　to let the oppressed go free,
to proclaim the year of the Lord's favor."

Luke 4:18–19 NRSV

Being Christian is as much a part of who Stephen Ministers are as eye color or body type is. Stephen Ministers carry their Christian faith with them, but this does not mean they try to force their faith on others. Rather, being Christian is what gives Stephen Ministers the desire to serve and the strength to hang in there with another through thick and thin—especially through thin. (There are usually plenty of people willing to be with another who is experiencing the thick parts of life: its goodness and abundance.)

From the Holy Spirit Stephen Ministers gain both the desire and the ability to be Christ to others: to walk with and love those who are hurting. As Stephen Ministers care, they rely on Christ; they know their own knowledge, experiences, or abilities are not enough to bring healing and wholeness to a care receiver.

Stephen Ministers' motivation for caring is not simply to "be nice." Their motivation for caring is described by the apostle Paul:

> Blessed be the God and Father of our Lord Jesus Christ, the Father of mercies and the God of all consolation, who consoles us in all our affliction, so that we may be able to console those who are in any affliction with the consolation with which we ourselves are consoled by God. For just as the sufferings of Christ are abundant for us, so also our consolation is abundant through Christ.
>
> 2 Corinthians 1:3–5 NRSV

Stephen Ministers want to bring their care receivers the same comfort and care that they themselves have received from "the God of all consolation."

Recruited and Selected Caregivers

To ensure that Stephen Ministers have the necessary gifts, interest, and commitment, congregations recruit candidates and then carefully select them based on their character and qualifications. Stephen Leaders interview all who are interested in being Stephen Ministers. The goal of these interviews is to help both the Stephen Leaders and the candidates learn whether Stephen Ministry is right for the applicants, in keeping with who they are and what God has called them to do. People with the necessary gifts, interest, and commitment for Stephen Ministry are recruited to take the training class. When the selecting is properly done, people who can't maintain confidentiality will be screened out. People who believe they themselves can straighten out someone else's life will not be invited to become involved. People who are drawn to Stephen Ministry because they themselves are hurting and want their own needs met will be helped to find the care they need and perhaps invited to reapply at a later time.

Trained and Commissioned Caregivers

Stephen Ministers receive thorough training to prepare them for their caregiving ministry. After individuals satisfactorily complete their 50 hours of initial training, they are commissioned by their congregation as Stephen Ministers and assigned to care receivers. This commissioning serves as the formal acceptance and validation of these caregivers by the congregation. While they are actively serving, whether with or without caregiving relationships, Stephen Ministers participate in twice-monthly supervision and continuing education.

The goal of training and of commissioning is not to declare that Stephen Ministers have been made over into experts or professionals. The goal is, first, to help them become competent as distinctively Christian lay caregivers, and second, to secure the congregation's affirmation of this competence.

Supervised Caregivers

Stephen Ministers are not left to perform their caring ministry alone—they participate in Small Group Peer Supervision twice each month. Supervision takes place in small groups (usually five to seven Stephen Ministers) led by a Supervision Group Facilitator, who is a Stephen Leader or a Stephen Minister with additional training in group facilitation skills. In supervision Stephen Ministers report on and explore their caring relationships in a structured setting that offers support and encouragement, and that holds them accountable. They do this in a manner that protects the confidentiality of care receivers.

In addition to the support Stephen Ministers receive from one another in supervision, they also depend on support from their Stephen Leaders, their congregation, and their pastors. Stephen Leaders are available for advice and help. Congregation members pray for Stephen Ministry and refer friends and family in need of lay caregiving to the congregation's Stephen Ministry. Pastors cast a compelling vision for Stephen Ministry, encourage individuals to receive care from Stephen Ministers, and offer guidance and encouragement to Stephen Ministers in challenging caregiving situations. Pastors also help the congregation understand how Stephen Ministry is part of their fulfillment of Jesus' command to love one another.

Who Stephen Ministers Are Not

The preceding information yields insights into who Stephen Ministers are. To understand more fully their role as lay Christian caregivers, it helps to consider who they are not. Stephen Ministers are not professional caregivers, and they do not serve as or replace any of the following types of caregivers.

Not Pastors

All Christians are ministers, but only some are pastors. The pastor is the shepherd and spiritual leader of a congregation, although he or she may sometimes serve in a more specialized role, such as hospital or military chaplain, staff person at a social service agency, or professor at a seminary. While the caring that Stephen Ministers do is somewhat similar to pastoral care, pastors do many other kinds of ministry as well. Therefore, congregations should not call Stephen Ministers "lay pastors." Such a label risks projecting expectations onto Stephen Ministers that they are not gifted, trained, or called to fulfill.

Not Therapists or Counselors

Stephen Ministers are not therapists or counselors. They are trained to do some activities that are similar to those counselors do, such as listening reflectively, expressing empathy, demonstrating assertiveness, and dealing with feelings. Doing these activities, however, does not make them counselors. Caring parents and effective supervisors also know and practice these skills. All healthy relationships include these basic dynamics.

While there are a few surface similarities between what Stephen Ministers and mental health professionals do, one need not go very deep to find major differences. Stephen

Ministers are not qualified to diagnose mental or emotional disturbances, while mental health professionals need to be competent in this area. Therapists and counselors address issues that Stephen Ministers are not equipped to handle, such as problems with active addictions, psychosis, suicidal situations, eating disorders, and medication assessment and management. Given the expectations that people have of counselors and therapists, congregations should not describe Stephen Ministers as "lay counselors" or "lay therapists."

Not Spiritual Directors

While quality Christian care often promotes spiritual growth, Stephen Ministers are not spiritual directors. Spiritual director is a formal title earned by a person who has been called and trained to guide people into a closer walk with Christ through an intense, focused, one-to-one process of directed spiritual growth.

Individuals who need the care of a Stephen Minister have different needs from those who seek the help of a spiritual director. Stephen Ministry care receivers usually have as their principal issue some life crisis or challenge. Certainly the care receiver's relationship with Christ will be strengthened and grow deeper as a result of his or her time with a Stephen Minister, but the hoped-for outcome is healing and relief from a set of emotional struggles.

In contrast, the primary goal of those seeking the assistance of a spiritual director is a quest for spiritual growth. During this quest a person's daily life will be affected, but this is a secondary effect of his or her faith journey. If a person primarily wants to further his or her Christian discipleship through being mentored, he or she needs a spiritual director, not a Stephen Minister.

Not Peers in Recovery

There are many outstanding self-help groups that help their members recover from various traumas, such as childhood abuse or alcoholism. Everyone in such a group shares a particular life challenge. For example, everyone in a recovery group for incest survivors is an incest survivor; everyone in a Narcotics Anonymous group is recovering from chemical dependency. But Stephen Ministers are different. Even though they have never had cancer, for example, they can still care for someone who is fighting cancer.

Not Best Friends

A Stephen Minister is not a care receiver's best friend. While some characteristics of the Stephen Ministry relationship are similar to those in a friendship, there is a key difference: The Stephen Ministry relationship is designed to focus on the care receiver's needs. The Stephen Minister does not expect to be able to talk about his or her concerns as well as listen to the care receiver's, as would happen in a friendship. For another example, a care receiver is not likely to drop by a Stephen Minister's house unexpectedly and say, "Hi, I was just in the neighborhood and thought I'd drop by to see if you want to go to a movie." If the care receiver does this, the Stephen Minister will almost certainly assertively decline the invitation in order clearly to communicate appropriate, crucial boundaries in the caregiving relationship.

A Stephen Minister could certainly offer support to a care receiver who has moved into town following the death of a spouse, for example, and who is now ready to make new friends. The Stephen Minister would encourage the care receiver in his or her search for new close friends, but the Stephen Minister would not fill that role him- or herself.

Not Independent Caregivers

Stephen Ministers are not lone rangers. They do not seek out and establish Stephen Ministry relationships on their own. They receive assignments from their Referrals Coordinator—a Stephen Leader or pastor who meets with potential care receivers to determine whether a Stephen Minister can meet their needs. Stephen Ministers show their interdependence by their faithful participation in Small Group Peer Supervision. Whether or not they are currently serving a care receiver, Stephen Ministers participate regularly in supervision. A Stephen Minister who goes on sabbatical, resigns, or retires must formally close any caring relationship he or she is involved with.

The Value of Understanding Who Stephen Ministers Are

Understanding who Stephen Ministers are and the boundaries of the Stephen Ministry relationship can help Stephen Leaders, pastors, mental health professionals, and others effectively consider Stephen Ministry as an option for care. When you who are training to be Stephen Ministers know your role and how it fits with the responsibilities of other caring professionals, you can more easily recognize situations for which you are not trained. Should such instances occur, you will be equipped to alert your Stephen Leaders or pastors so that a care receiver's needs can be effectively addressed by the appropriate professional resource.

2

What Stephen Ministers Do and Do Not Do

Henry's wife, Inez, died after they had been married for 37 years. Henry could hardly remember what life had been like before he got married, so he couldn't imagine how he was going to get by without Inez. He could manage the cooking and cleaning—that was no problem. He just didn't know how he was going to deal with the loneliness.

Soon after the funeral Pastor Garcia offered to arrange for a Stephen Minister to visit with Henry. Henry said yes immediately. He knew he needed someone to talk with as he tried to sort out life without Inez.

Rick, Henry's Stephen Minister, visited a couple of days later. Rick explained a little about what a Stephen Ministry relationship was like and then sat back and listened. At first, Henry was reluctant to talk much about what he was really feeling. He found it hard to talk about such things with a stranger. After a couple of visits, however, Rick seemed more like a trusted friend. When Henry talked about his feelings, Rick asked questions that made it easier for him to talk even more freely. When Henry cried he felt embarrassed, but Rick's calm acceptance helped him get over his embarrassment quickly. When Henry wondered if there were others recently widowed with whom he could talk, Rick helped him find a support group. When Henry wanted to talk about whether Inez was in heaven, Rick carefully listened to Henry's questions and fears and then reassured Henry with words from the Bible. When they first started meeting, Rick would offer a prayer at the beginning and end of the visit. Over time Henry became more comfortable with praying with another person and they each would pray aloud at times.

Rick visited Henry almost every week for a year and a half. By that time Henry had made his peace with Inez's death. He still missed her, but he had started looking forward to and planning for the rest of his life. About that time Rick gently suggested that the time was approaching when Henry wouldn't need the caring relationship any longer. At first Henry was shocked and said he wasn't ready for that, but as they talked about it Henry realized that Rick was right. He would always be thankful for Rick's ministry, and they remained friends, but Henry's need for a Stephen Ministry relationship had ended.

What Stephen Ministers Do

The introductory vignette illustrates some of the activities that characterize Stephen Ministry. Following are more complete descriptions of what you will be doing when you are a Stephen Minister.

Stephen Ministers Care

The best way to describe what Stephen Ministers do is to say that they care; they "Bear one another's burdens, and in this way . . . fulfill the law of Christ" (Galatians 6:2 NRSV). Stephen Ministers usually meet with their care receivers in person once a week for about an hour, and they may also talk with their care receivers over the telephone occasionally, depending on the needs of the situation and the point in the caring relationship. They listen to their care receivers, help them recognize and express their feelings, maintain appropriate boundaries, and remain committed to their care receivers over the long haul. Stephen Ministers maintain their care receivers' confidentiality. They don't try to solve others' problems but rather help others work through their own problems.

Stephen Ministers know their own limitations, and when they find that their care receivers have needs for which they aren't qualified to care, they work with their Supervision Group, Stephen Leaders, and pastor to refer their care receivers to mental health professionals or other more qualified caregivers. When their care receivers no longer need their caring relationships, Stephen Ministers bring closure and move on to another ministry assignment.

Distinctively Christian Care

A defining characteristic of Stephen Ministers' care is that it is distinctively Christian. Stephen Ministers care as God's servants. They count on God's power to bring about healing and hope. Stephen Ministers also use the powerful caring tools of the Christian faith: prayer, the Bible, confession and forgiveness, blessings, and "a cup of cold water" for those who are thirsty (Matthew 10:42), which is a metaphor for providing concrete, practical care when that's what people need.[1] Stephen Ministers are trained to use these powerful caring tools carefully and appropriately, which is to say, to use them to meet care receivers' needs, not their own, and to listen before and after using distinctively Christian caring resources.

1 These distinctively Christian caring tools are explained in *Christian Caregiving— a Way of Life* by Kenneth C. Haugk (St. Louis: Stephen Ministries, 2012).

Jesus said, "'A new command I give you: Love one another. As I have loved you, so you must love one another. By this all men will know that you are my disciples, if you love one another'" (John 13:34–35). Paul wrote to the Galatians, "Carry each other's burdens, and in this way you will fulfill the law of Christ" (Galatians 6:2). These verses help define what Stephen Ministers do. They care because Jesus told them to and they try to care as he did. Their care is an expression of Christian community in which God's children share the challenges that life brings and also share the love that Jesus both commanded and made possible. While the instructions in these verses apply to all Christians, Stephen Ministers are specially gifted, trained, and sent out to provide such Christian care to those in need on behalf of the entire congregation.

Stephen Ministers on the Continuum of Care

The care that Stephen Ministers provide is somewhere between the care that an acquaintance or friend would provide and the care people would receive from a pastor or a

Informal Caring		Semiformal Caring		Formal Caring
Casual Acquaintance	Close Friend	Stephen Minister	Pastor	Therapist or Counselor

Fig. 1. Continuum of Care

mental health professional. The Continuum of Care in Figure 1 illustrates the fact that Stephen Ministry is more formal than the care an acquaintance or a friend provides because it is structured and focuses on the care receiver's needs. It is less formal, however, than the care that pastors or mental health professionals provide. These professional caregivers, with their greater training and experience and their particular orientation, explore care receivers' needs at deeper levels than Stephen Ministers do. In addition, mental health professionals usually formalize the caring relationship by receiving payment for their services. Stephen Ministers accept no payment for their voluntary caring ministry.

Kinds of Needs Stephen Ministers Care For

Stephen Ministers provide spiritual and emotional one-to-one care to adults undergoing a wide variety of challenges or difficulties. Following are some of the needs that might typically call for Stephen Ministry.

Stephen Ministers care for persons who are:

- Bereaved
- Terminally ill
- Separated or divorcing
- Hospitalized or convalescing
- Single parents
- Experiencing vocational stresses, such as relocation, reorganization, termination, or starting a new job
- Refugees
- Students living away from home
- Residents of long-term care facilities
- Inmates of jails, prisons, or detention centers
- Caretakers of ill or disabled persons
- Adjusting to family changes such as remarriage, institutionalization of a family member, or a new baby
- Parents whose children present exceptional challenges
- Newlyweds
- Homebound
- Coping with infertility
- Entering or reentering the job market
- Retiring
- Dealing with adoption issues

- Victims of crime
- New residents of a community
- Preparing for professional Christian service
- Chronically ill, in pain, or disabled
- Survivors of natural disasters or other catastrophes
- In the military

Five Types of Care

Stephen Ministers may provide five types of care: crisis care, follow-up care, chronic care, preventive care, and caregiver care.

1. Crisis Care

Stephen Ministers often help people cope with life crises such as hospitalization, terminal illness, the death of a loved one, unemployment, or a natural disaster. Crises can throw people into a tailspin. Coping mechanisms that worked in the past don't work as well in the face of the crisis. People in crisis can benefit greatly from a Stephen Minister's compassionate, objective care.

Sometimes Stephen Ministers become involved in caring for people immediately after the onset of a crisis. One possible strategy is for a pastor, with the potential care receiver's permission, to take a Stephen Minister along the first time he or she visits after a crisis, such as an unexpected death. This allows the care receiver to be introduced to the Stephen Minister by a trusted pastor. The pastor can offer Stephen Ministry to the care receiver soon thereafter, in a private visit.

To the Stephen Leader

This changes the sequence of events for referrals slightly, but you can see how it could be incorporated in that process.

Pastors need to discern carefully which situations are appropriate for a Stephen Minister to accompany them. Inappropriate circumstances would include situations where sensitive information may be shared. In those situations, the pastor can meet with the person in crisis privately and present Stephen Ministry as a possibility.

Once a Stephen Minister has been assigned to the care receiver in crisis, one option is for the pastor and the Stephen Minister both to continue to meet regularly with the care receiver for a while, although at different times. Over time the frequency of the pastor's visits would drop off, based on the care receiver's needs and the other demands on the pastor's time. But the Stephen Minister will continue meeting regularly with the care receiver until the care receiver no longer needs the Stephen Minister's care.

2. Follow-Up Care

Externally it may seem as though a crisis is over and done with in a matter of days or, at most, weeks. But for people experiencing that crisis, the initial topsy-turvy time is just the beginning of what will continue for some time. Much work remains for them. In this follow-up period, Stephen Ministers have a unique role of caregiving to play, one not easily met by any other caregiving the congregation might offer.

Many pastors are acutely aware of the need for follow-up care and have been trained to understand its importance. Howard Clinebell's *Basic Types of Pastoral Care and Counseling* stresses this need.

When death or any severe loss strikes, the usual response is feelings of psychological numbness and shock (nature's anesthesia) mixed with feelings of unreality—of being in a nightmare from which one expects to awaken. The mind cannot yet accept the overwhelming pain—the reality that the person is really gone. Accepting the full reality of the loss must eventually occur or the healing will be incomplete. This acceptance must occur gradually, usually over a period of months.[2]

Knowing the crucial importance of follow-up care places pastors in a bind. They often go from one crisis to the next with little or no time to provide adequate follow-up care. Their role is similar to that of firefighters who put out the flames at one fire but then must leave to fight the next blaze. Stephen Ministers, however, stick with the care receivers, help them sort through the emotional ashes, and care faithfully as care receivers go about rebuilding their lives.

3. Chronic Care

Stephen Ministers occasionally care for people experiencing long-term disabilities such as chronic pain or a degenerative disease. Often a care receiver in this situation also receives care from physicians, nurses, physical therapists, family, friends, clergy, and others. Stephen Ministers fill an important place in the overall plan for care. They listen to the care receiver, pray with him or her, value what the care receiver feels and thinks, and help connect him or her to the outside world.

When Stephen Ministers provide care to a chronically ill person, however, they are ministering to a care receiver whose situation is unlikely to change. A compassionate Stephen Minister enters into the care receiver's situation, to an extent, and shares his or her pain and frustration. This can pose a special challenge to Stephen Ministers. They rely on their Supervision Groups to provide the support

2 Howard Clinebell, *Basic Types of Pastoral Care and Counseling: Resources for the Ministry of Healing and Growth*, rev. ed. (Nashville: Abingdon Press, 1984), p. 222.

and encouragement they need to keep going. In some chronic care situations, both the care receiver and the Stephen Minister may benefit if a new Stephen Minister is assigned every year or so.

4. Preventive Care

Certain life events may unexpectedly throw people into crises.

A couple whose youngest child is going off to college may be looking forward to new freedom, but when the child leaves they find themselves sad and lonely.

A person moves into town and at first seems to be coping with the change well, but after a few weeks shows signs of being lonely and depressed.

A man has worked hard all his life and been very successful, and now he is looking forward to his retirement as a time to enjoy the fruit of his labor. After he retires, however, he finds his life empty, meaningless, and boring.

A couple is excited and happy about their soon-to-be-born child. After the birth, however, the realities of day-to-day parenting leave one spouse sometimes frustrated and missing the life she used to have.

While such crises may surprise care receivers, it is sometimes possible to see the crises coming and prevent them, or minister to the person very early on and reduce the negative impact of the circumstance. That is the purpose of preventive care. When a change is anticipated, the pastor may talk to the person, letting him or her know that any change, no matter how wanted it may be, can produce stress. The pastor can assess the person's receptivity—now or in the future—to a Stephen Minister.

Stephen Ministers can help care receivers prepare for the emotional turmoil that a major life change can bring. In other instances, a pastor or someone else close to an individual may detect early signs of a beginning downward spiral as a result of a change in circumstances. A Stephen Minister might be assigned to a parent whose nest will soon be empty, for example, or where the child has recently left. The Stephen Minister can help the care receiver think about the future or share about how he or she feels now that the child is gone. This could nip in the bud a developing sadness. The Stephen Minister would continue to care, listening as the care receiver shares feelings and helping the care receiver think through the adjustments he or she needs to make.

Some caring relationships that focus on preventive care may last only a month or two; that may be all it takes for the care receiver to see the upcoming challenge and make the necessary adjustments. Other caring relationships that begin as preventive care may last for months or longer.

5. Caregiver Care

Stephen Ministers can offer valuable support to those who are behind the scenes caring for someone else in crisis, but who themselves also need care. Lending care to a caregiver strengthens that person to continue providing support. This is indeed sharing one another's burdens. Here are a few examples.

A young adult is disabled in an automobile accident and has to live with his parents because he is unable to care for himself. His mother's life is turned upside down by the demands of caring for her son, and she needs a Stephen Minister to listen as she expresses and deals with strong feelings.

A man's parents divorce after 38 years of marriage. Both his mother and his father turn to him for understanding and support. Meanwhile he has his own grief and anger to deal with, and a Stephen Minister will help him do so.

An elderly woman cares for her husband over time as his advancing Alzheimer's disease puts more and more burdens on her. A succession of Stephen Ministers helps her cope and survive.

Caregiver care refers to caring for those who are caregivers, supporting them in their need. The Stephen Minister provides an ear for them, a nonjudging listener who can share their frustrations and fears, weariness and wishes. The Stephen Minister may also be a go-between to help the individual get respite through other caring offerings of the congregation or the community.

What Stephen Ministers Do Not Do

It is equally important to understand the types of care that Stephen Ministers do not provide.

Types of Care Stephen Ministers Do Not Provide

Stephen Ministers do not serve as caregivers for:
- Minors

- Couples, families, or other groups
- Those who are suffering serious mental or emotional disturbances
- Those suffering severe depression
- Those with personality disorders
- Manipulative individuals
- Those dealing with abuse issues
- Substance abusers or chemically dependent persons
- Those exhibiting suicidal behavior
- Those exhibiting violent behavior

Pastors, Stephen Leaders, and Stephen Ministers do not diagnose mental health disorders, but they can learn to recognize some of the symptoms and behaviors that might indicate a care receiver's need for a mental health professional. Following are some situations in which a Referrals Coordinator should not refer a potential care receiver to a Stephen Minister since these situations are not appropriate for Stephen Ministry.

Some of these situations may also develop as an already-existing caring relationship goes on, or they may not have been evident at the time of referral. If they become evident during your caring relationship, you as the Stephen Minister need to discuss the situation with

To the Mental Health Professional

Note that in the Stephen Series system the word *referral* has two very different meanings. One is the process of identifying care receivers, preparing them, and linking them with Stephen Ministers—usually referred to in the plural as *referrals*. The other meaning is the one that this book explains: referring care receivers to a mental health professional or other caring resource.

your Supervision Group and one or more Stephen Leaders. Then you would talk to the care receiver about the need for a mental health professional's care. (Chapter 6 tells you how to conduct this talk.)

Stephen Ministers Do Not Serve as Caregivers for Minors

There are several good reasons why Stephen Leaders do not assign Stephen Ministers to work with minors. First, minors cannot give legal consent to receive care from a Stephen Minister. Second, since parents have a legal right to know what is said and done in any caring relationship where their child is the care receiver, it would be difficult to guarantee confidentiality in the caring relationship. Finally, there's always the worry about the potential for abuse of minors and about the vulnerability of minors as care receivers. Given these concerns, Stephen Ministers caring for minors could compromise a congregation's Stephen Ministry and greatly increase the potential for liability problems. It is best to refer minors to more appropriate caregivers.

Stephen Ministers Do Not Serve as Caregivers for Couples, Families, or Other Groups

Stephen Ministers work one-to-one with assigned care receivers. They do not work with couples, parents and children, or with other pairs or groups. The dynamics of working with more than one person conjointly are considerably more complex than working one-to-one. Such work is beyond the training of a Stephen Minister.

Although a Stephen Minister may work with a care receiver who has experienced a divorce or other family crisis, a Stephen Minister is not a marriage counselor or family therapist. Consequently, when dealing with care receivers who are experiencing difficulties in relationships, the

Stephen Minister's role would be to care for an individual, not to work with all parties involved. If another family member needs Stephen Ministry, perhaps Stephen Leaders can assign another Stephen Minister to him or her.

Stephen Ministers Do Not Serve as Caregivers for Those Suffering Serious Mental or Emotional Disturbance

Sometimes people in crisis suffer deep emotional turmoil. If a care receiver experiences severe mental or emotional disturbances, the Stephen Leader needs to work with the Stephen Minister to refer that care receiver immediately to an appropriate mental health professional.

Indicators that more in-depth care is needed include grossly abnormal behaviors such as hallucinating, excessive talking to oneself, or complete withdrawal from others. Further indicators may include paranoid behavior, manifested in delusions of persecution or delusions of grandeur. Mentally or emotionally disturbed persons may exhibit sharp mood swings or show excessive anger, sadness, or hostility. When people are unable to perform basic life functions such as keeping themselves or their homes clean, adhering to a time schedule, sleeping or eating normally, going to work, or making simple decisions, they clearly need more help than Stephen Ministers can give; they need to be referred, many times with some urgency, to mental health professionals.

Stephen Ministers Do Not Serve as Caregivers for Those Suffering Severe Depression

One in five persons suffers from severe depression at some point in his or her life. The symptoms include weight loss or gain, persistent lack of sleep or excessive sleep, loss of sexual desire, lack of self-esteem, unexplained aches or pains, a loss of interest in previously enjoyed activities or relationships, and other ongoing difficulties at home or at work.

According to one definition, there are three types of depression.

- *Mild depression* is the most common and can be brought on by both happy and sad events. For example, a wedding certainly is a happy time, but it is also very stressful, and the stress can cause depression. Another common cause of depression is childbirth, which may lead to postpartum blues for the mother.

- *Moderate depression*, or a feeling of hopelessness, lasts longer and is more intense. It is often brought on by a sad event, such as the death of a loved one or loss of a job. It usually does not interfere with daily living. If it persists, professional help may be warranted.

- *Severe depression* can cause a person to lose interest in the outside world, can disrupt everyday life, and can lead to suicide. A person with severe depression experiences some of the previously named symptoms to a profound degree and needs professional treatment.[3]

According to the above definitions, Stephen Ministers can minister effectively to persons experiencing mild depression (with the caution that such depression may deepen). Stephen Ministry may also be appropriate for some persons with moderate depression caused by situations like the death of a loved one or a negative medical report. If the person's symptoms persist or worsen and begin to disrupt his or her daily life (for example, an inability to sleep, failure to maintain personal hygiene), then the individual requires professional assistance, or at least a professional evaluation.

3 Reprinted with permission of the Missouri Department of Mental Health, Division of Comprehensive Psychiatric Services, P.O. Box 687, 1706 East Elm, Jefferson City, MO 65102, (573) 751-8017. Sponsored by the Missouri Advisory Council for Comprehensive Psychiatric Services.

Stephen Ministers Do Not Serve as Caregivers for Those with Personality Disorders

Some people find it very difficult to relate to others or cope with life. They may have deep-seated and persistent psychological problems known as personality disorders. According to a widely accepted understanding of personality disorders:

> Patients with personality disorders show deeply ingrained, inflexible, and maladaptive patterns of relating to and perceiving both the environment and themselves. . . . Because such persons do not routinely acknowledge pain from what society perceives as their symptoms, they are often regarded as unmotivated for treatment and impervious to recovery.[4]

Some examples of personality disorders include obsessive-compulsive personality, histrionic personality, and antisocial personality. Personality disorders vary greatly in severity, and many persons with them work very hard in treatment. Such individuals need the care that professionals can offer. Stephen Ministers are not qualified to give them the care they need.

Stephen Ministers Do Not Serve as Caregivers for Manipulative Individuals

Manipulative or controlling behavior often causes difficulties in a variety of relationships. Everett L. Shostrom describes manipulators as more deceitful, controlling, and cynical. Nonmanipulators, he says, are more honest, aware, free, and trusting.[5]

A portrait of a manipulator is found in John 12:1–8.

4 Harold I. Kaplan, Benjamin J. Sadock, and Jack A. Grebb, *Kaplan and Sadock's Synopsis of Psychiatry: Behavioral Sciences, Clinical Psychiatry*, Seventh Edition (Baltimore: Williams and Wilkins, 1994), p. 731.

5 Everett L. Shostrom, *Man the Manipulator: The Inner Journey from Manipulation to Actualization* (Nashville: Abingdon Press, 1967), pp. 50–51.

When Mary anoints Jesus' feet with costly perfume and wipes them with her hair, Judas says, "'Why was this perfume not sold for three hundred denarii and the money given to the poor?'" The Gospel writer goes on to report, "He said this not because he cared about the poor, but because he was a thief; he kept the common purse and used to steal what was put into it" (John 12:5–6 NRSV). Judas exhibits the signs of a manipulator: He has deceitful motives. His tunnel vision makes him unaware of the important issues of life. Judas attempts to control others by using guilt and shame. He is cynically immune to the beautiful act of ministry that Mary performs.

Manipulative individuals often make completely inappropriate demands that quickly test the skill and patience of those who attempt to care for them. You may spot manipulative behavior in your first conversations with an individual. Others, however, may manipulate so smoothly that you are unaware of it for quite some time. Since even experienced pastors and trained professional caregivers have difficulty dealing with manipulative persons, such care receivers are certainly too demanding for any Stephen Minister. Even though a manipulator may not act on a recommendation to receive care from a mental health professional, such a referral is definitely the correct action for a Stephen Leader or Stephen Minister to take.

Stephen Ministers Do Not Serve as Caregivers for Those Dealing with Abuse Issues

A person experiencing abuse, or inflicting it, or needing to heal from past abuse, needs a referral to the proper authorities and other community resources. Abuse does not fall within the bounds of an appropriate Stephen Ministry caring relationship. If such information is revealed during a caring relationship, the Stephen Minister will talk to a

Stephen Leader, who in turn will bring in the pastor, an attorney, and a mental health professional for consultation.

A Stephen Minister who learns that a care receiver is a victim or a perpetrator of sexual abuse may be required by law to report that information. The laws concerning various types of abuse—child, spouse, or elder—vary by state. They also may change from year to year within a given state. It is essential, therefore, to consult an attorney and a mental health professional before making a report or deciding you don't need to do so. This will also ensure that your report, if needed, follows the proper procedures and will help protect everyone involved.

The measured process described here means a Stephen Minister and a Stephen Leader can operate with a bias toward reporting. Be alert to possibilities of abuse. If danger to another person seems imminent, do not leave the person until the proper authorities have shown up. Given the possibilities for delay (for example, your congregation's attorney is out of town or the mental health professional you ordinarily use is in an all-day meeting), take whatever steps you must to get help in a timely manner.

Stephen Ministers Do Not Serve as Caregivers for Those Struggling with Substance Abuse, Chemical Dependency, or Other Addictions

Specialists in the mental health field and members of 12-step programs (e.g., Alcoholics Anonymous, Narcotics Anonymous) are best equipped to help individuals who abuse drugs, alcohol, or other substances, as well as those struggling with other addictions such as gambling or pornography. Symptoms such as alcohol on a person's breath early in the day, inappropriate or unnaturally elevated moods, slow physical reactions, slurred speech, and chronic absenteeism from work or school may indicate the need to involve a specialist. To find a specialist, call the published number of the relevant 12-step program, or contact a mental health professional for references. Stephen Ministers are not trained to work with persons struggling with substance abuse or other addictions.

Stephen Ministers Do Not Serve as Caregivers for Those Exhibiting Suicidal Behavior

Any mention of suicide must be considered a serious threat. When an individual talks about suicide, many unspoken thoughts are behind those words. Here are some variables to look for in order to assess suicide risk.

- *Symptoms of depression.* A disproportionately large number of those who are severely depressed attempt suicide.

- *Previous threats.* A history of suicide threats is a sign to caregivers that the person has an increased likelihood of an actual attempt.

- *Previous attempts.* A person who has attempted suicide is at high risk, even if the attempts were not too serious. A high percentage of those who take their own lives have made previous attempts.

- *Specific plans.* If an individual gives information about where, when, and how he or she intends to proceed with a plan for committing suicide, this is an extremely serious situation. For example, if the person says: "I'm going home this afternoon and take out my father's pistol, load it, and shoot myself in the heart," then the person is at very high risk.

- *Availability of means.* If the means are easily available, the risk increases sharply. A person who has immediate access to pills, guns, or a noose, for example, is at much higher risk than a person with no such access.

- *Lethality of means.* The risk for a person who intends to commit suicide by taking all the aspirins in a bottle is not as great as for someone who plans to jump off a high bridge into a river. Any person who wants to hurt him- or herself with any means needs professional care, but the more lethal the means that the person intends to use, the higher the risk.

- *Suicide-oriented actions.* If a person has prepared for the suicide attempt by such actions as making out a will, writing a suicide note or a letter to loved ones, buying a gun, or arranging a trip alone to an isolated camp, then that person is at a very high risk.

If there is a chance that the care receiver could be at risk to commit suicide, do not hesitate to seek immediate assistance, following the process you learned (or will learn) in Stephen Ministry training module 14, "Helping Suicidal Persons Get the Help They Need." In high-risk situations, call the police and do not leave the care receiver alone. All caregivers are advised to be safe rather than sorry.

Stephen Ministers Do Not Care for Someone Exhibiting Violent Behavior

If an individual behaves violently toward him- or herself or others, Stephen Leaders or Stephen Ministers should immediately refer him or her to a mental health professional or call the police. Don't wait; take action immediately.

Violent behavior includes abusive and suicidal behavior, self-mutilation, or threats to others. In such instances you may need to contact the police or a social services agency first. Then you may be able to assist the care receiver in getting help from a mental health professional.

Public and private agencies exist to help those dealing with all forms of violence. As part of the resources of

Stephen Ministry—chiefly in the *Community Resources Handbook* developed by your congregation's Stephen Ministry—this information will be available to you. Study it so you will know where to turn in an emergency.

Stephen Ministers Need to Refer When There Are Medical or Physical Problems

Sometimes physical problems signal a need for mental health assistance. For instance, loss of appetite, malnourishment, and dizziness can result from emotional difficulties. On the other hand, these and other physical symptoms may indicate a physical problem that needs medical attention. In any case, referring an individual with such symptoms to a medical professional is the place to begin.

An Issue of Boundaries

Boundaries are important factors in all relationships. They allow understanding about where one person's capabilities and responsibilities end and another's begin.

Stephen Ministers have a role to play in helping others through typical life crises. Mental health professionals need to provide the care when the need is serious. Knowing and respecting the boundaries between what Stephen Ministers do and what professionals do is a key to promoting quality care.

Stephen Ministers are not expected to handle challenging caring situations alone. There are support systems for these types of situations. The rest of this book provides more details about the support available to you.

3

Self-Help Groups

There are a growing number of self-help groups organized on the principle that people who share a common problem can band together to provide mutual support and to promote positive change. Although not professional in the strict sense of the term, they are a valuable and an effective part of the treatment landscape, often working very closely with mental health professionals and receiving referrals from them.

Stephen Ministers may make referrals to self-help groups in some circumstances. Although there is a wide variety of self-help groups, for your purposes as a Stephen Minister you will be chiefly concerned with four types.

Four Types of Self-Help Groups

1. Groups for chronic mental or physical conditions: for people with schizophrenia or diabetes, for example

2. Groups for caregivers of those who suffer from chronic mental or physical conditions

3. Groups for persons experiencing life's tragedies; for example, a group of people who have lost a child to Sudden Infant Death Syndrome (SIDS)

4. Groups for people with compulsions or addictions, such as Alcoholics Anonymous (AA)

For all these groups the principle that gathers people together is the same: Persons who have experienced or are experiencing the same situation or the same condition are better able to offer encouragement, support, and sometimes advice than those who have not experienced it. This principle holds up under study. Diabetics who meet with other diabetics do better than those who don't;[1] addicts who took part in a self-help group were less likely to revert to substance abuse;[2] breast cancer sufferers in a support group have double the survival rate of those who do not participate in such a group.[3]

Literally hundreds of local, state, and national self-help associations are organized around every issue from chemical addiction to compulsive shopping. These associations provide resources for hundreds of thousands of individuals who meet regularly for support and encouragement.

It is safe to assume that nearly every congregation has members who are using, or have used, self-help groups to help them deal with certain life issues. Many congregations also provide space for self-help groups to meet.

---

1 Janice L. Gilden, M.D., et al., "Diabetes Support Groups Improve Health Care of Older Diabetic Patients," *Journal of the American Geriatrics Society* 40, 2 (February 1992), 147–150.

2 James R. McKay et al., "Treatment Goals, Continuity of Care, and Outcome in a Day Hospital Substance Abuse Rehabilitation Program," *The American Journal of Psychiatry* 151, 2 (February 1994), 254–259.

3 David Spiegel, M.D., et al., "Effect of Psychosocial Treatment on Survival of Patients with Metastatic Breast Cancer," *The Lancet* 8668, 2 (1989), 888–891.

Four Types of Self-Help Groups

This section will present a closer look at the four different types of self-help groups that may be of value for your care receiver.

Self-Help Groups for Those with Mental or Physical Conditions

Life-threatening illnesses (cancer is an example) and chronic illnesses pose major challenges to people's well-being. Whether the diagnosis is breast cancer, diabetes, or schizophrenia, someone's life is changed markedly; and so is that of his or her family. Their vision of the future may be altered dramatically. What once was taken for granted may be thrown into terrible uncertainty.

Persons with a new diagnosis of a mental or physical illness find themselves identifying with a new group of peers made up of persons who are also dealing with "it," whatever it is. Often they want to hear from others who have been dealing longer with the problem and who can speak from intensely personal experience. It is natural, then, that groups would form around specific diagnoses. A few samples of such groups illustrate the type.

• Children and Adults with Attention Deficit Disorder (CHADD)

• Anxiety Disorders Association of America

• Diabetes Support Group for Adults

Increasingly, such self-help groups are viewed by health care professionals as essential in the treatment, recovery, and support of persons with certain illnesses. These groups often meet in space provided by a treatment center and may very well have a health care professional as a consultant. Health care professionals routinely encourage patients to participate in such groups as a way of coping with the effects of the illness.

Self-Help Groups for Caregivers of Those Who Suffer from Chronic Mental or Physical Conditions

Family members and friends also will benefit strongly from attending self-help groups for support and information sharing. Health care professionals will frequently recommend this. The wear and tear of constant care for someone with Alzheimer's disease, for example, is made more bearable in the company of those who know what you are enduring. Local branches of the Alzheimer's Association provide a variety of support groups for caregivers.

Self-Help Groups for Persons Experiencing Life's Tragedies

Many people look for support through a self-help group when they are going through tragic changes in their lives. These changes may include experiences such as divorce, death of a spouse, or the loss of a baby through Sudden Infant Death Syndrome. The ability to share one's feelings and concerns with others who have gone through or are going through the same experience helps a person know that he or she is not alone. Other examples of such groups:

- Anencephaly Support Foundation—support for parents who elect to continue a pregnancy after a diagnosis of an anencephalic (having no brain) infant

- Compassionate Friends–support for parents whose children have died

- Mothers Against Drunk Driving (MADD)—some local MADD chapters offer support for family members or others who were close to those killed or injured by drunk drivers

• Parents without Partners—support for single parents

Because members of such groups are at different stages in processing their loss, newcomers can be reasonably confident of finding resources and strategies for dealing with the tragedy at the point where they are.

Self-Help Groups for People with Compulsions and Addictions

Millions of persons suffer from an inability to control independently some behavior that is distressing and destructive. Persons who join groups for those with compulsions or addictions have acknowledged their addiction and are seeking the group's help in resisting the behavior. The group is able to offer this help because its members understand the problem through personal experience. Together they have developed a group culture resilient enough to withstand the turmoil of helping someone alter long-standing, destructive behavior patterns.

Most of these groups base their approach on modifications of the Twelve Steps of Alcoholics Anonymous and are called "twelve-step groups." Groups are oriented toward specific issues such as narcotics abuse, overeating, sexual addiction, and other vexing problems.

There also are similar groups for the friends and loved ones of persons struggling with these issues. Al-Anon, a support program for those who are in relationship with an alcoholic, may be the most familiar of these groups. Other examples include:

• Alateen—support for teen-aged and young family members of alcoholics

• Gamblers Anonymous—support for compulsive gamblers

- Narcotics Anonymous—support for those abusing drugs

- Overeaters Anonymous—support for those with addictive eating habits

- Parents Anonymous—support for those at risk for abusing their children

The Best-Known Self-Help Group: Alcoholics Anonymous

The best-known self-help group is Alcoholics Anonymous, or AA, as it is often called. It has served as a prototype for more than one hundred kindred groups.

AA came into existence in 1935 in Akron, Ohio, as a result of the meeting of William Griffith Wilson, a former New York stockbroker, and Dr. Robert Holbrook Smith, an Akron surgeon. Both Bill W. and Dr. Bob, as they are often called in AA tradition, suffered the ravages of uncontrolled, addictive alcohol consumption. Both had lost much to their chemical dependency and stood on the edge of losing what they had left of family and livelihood. Both had tried everything they could imagine to stop, without success. They realized that by helping each other, they stood a chance to stop drinking before they died from their addiction.

Dr. Bob and Bill W. were successful. Their small beginning evolved into a movement that has helped hundreds of thousands of men and women find a way out of the morass of alcohol dependence. Their model for recovery, called the Twelve Steps, has been used and adapted by many self-help groups. The Twelve Steps of AA are:

1. We admitted we were powerless over alcohol—that our lives had become unmanageable.

2. Came to believe that a Power greater than ourselves could restore us to sanity.

3. Made a decision to turn our will and our lives over to the care of God *as we understood God*.

4. Made a searching and fearless moral inventory of ourselves.

5. Admitted to God, to ourselves, and to another human being the exact nature of our wrongs.

6. Were entirely ready to have God remove all these defects of character.

7. Humbly asked God to remove our shortcomings.

8. Made a list of all persons we had harmed, and became willing to make amends to them all.

9. Made direct amends to such people wherever possible, except when to do so would injure them or others.

10. Continued to take personal inventory and when we were wrong promptly admitted it.

11. Sought through prayer and meditation to improve our conscious contact with God *as we understood God*, praying only for knowledge of God's will for us and the power to carry that out.

12. Having had a spiritual awakening as the result of these steps, we tried to carry this message to alcoholics, and to practice these principles in all our affairs.[4]

Strengths of Self-Help Groups

Self-help groups offer many advantages to their members, not least of which is that they work for a lot of people.

---

4 "J," *A Simple Program: A Contemporary Translation of the Book* Alcoholics Anonymous (New York: Hyperion, 1996), pp. 55–56.

A few of the other key advantages follow, with most of them applying to all four types of self-help groups. Where the advantages are specifically related to twelve-step type groups, that will be indicated.

Community

Persons dealing with ravaging personal issues routinely think they are the only one in the entire world with such problems—until they meet some of the millions of fellow sufferers at a group meeting! Giving up the idea that one is uniquely cursed is one of the first blessings for many new members of self-help groups.

People with the sorts of personal problems that have given rise to self-help groups often feel a lot of shame. They think they are not living up to social expectations and surely must be terribly weak to be experiencing such difficulty and pain. A frequent sense of inferiority often causes them to pull back from others and become isolated from meaningful, supportive community. Self-help groups offer a new sense of community where members can discover a new and positive identity in relationship with others who are in the process of healing and growing. Persons arrive fearful and ashamed, are made welcome, and receive hope that life can get better. They learn that they do not have to struggle alone, that the group will be there for them. This can lead to a great deal of bonding or cohesiveness among self-help group members.

Economy

The price of admission to most self-help groups is a desire to get better. Rich or poor, insured or uninsured, all persons can come to a meeting based on their simple desire to get better. The "Foreword to the First Edition" of *Alcoholics Anonymous* describes the concept this way:

> We are not an organization in the conventional sense of the word. There are no fees or dues whatsoever. The only requirement for membership is a desire to stop drinking. We are not allied with any particular faith, sect, or denomination, nor do we oppose anyone. We simply wish to be helpful to those who are afflicted.[5]

While many participants in self-help groups may also benefit from professional care, whether medical or psychological, it is clear that many persons have profited from membership in such groups before, during, and after professional care. The free, or at least low-cost, nature of the assistance rendered by self-help groups makes it possible for almost everyone to participate and benefit.

Egalitarianism

Self-help groups typically are not hierarchical. No acknowledged pecking order separates one person from another. There may be a facilitator, but if the facilitator does her or his job well, each group member will be encouraged to provide support to the other members. The facilitator is not the "answer person" but rather someone to guide the conversation and address conflict when necessary. Distinctions among group members are nearly nonexistent. The person who has been sober for 30 years knows he or she is "one drink away from being drunk." Depending on their progress in dealing with an issue and their needs at that moment, group members will typically take turns being caregivers and care receivers, sometimes going back and forth between the two roles in the same meeting.

---

5 "J," *A Simple Program,* xvi.

Education

In many cases a self-help group is valuable in educating members about their particular disease, problem, or addiction. This education may focus on explaining why certain symptoms are occurring, suggesting simple steps that will help a person deal with the problem, and sharing information about the benefits of obtaining medical treatment or psychotherapy. Members may learn from the discussions at the group meetings or from reading materials recommended at meetings.

Responsibility for Self

People who participate in self-help groups tend to develop a greater sense of personal responsibility for their problems and their treatment. "I was the problem, I am the problem, and I will be the problem" is one common way this is expressed in the course of a twelve-step group meeting. Because most addictive persons deny their problem in order to escape personal responsibility for their compulsive behavior, breaking through denial to face reality is an extremely important step.

The emphasis on equality in self-help groups promotes acceptance of personal responsibility. Persons learn both the importance of self-reliance and of caring for others. Self-help groups involve the person in the treatment decisions. People assume responsibility for helping shape the course of the care they receive. Taking responsibility in this manner makes the person a partner with any professionals involved in his or her care instead of a passive object of treatment. This leads to a great deal of empowerment for the group member.

Self-reliance is a snare and a delusion for addictive persons, of course. "I drink; we stay sober" is one way this truth is expressed in AA meetings. Through the twelve steps the person suffering from chemical dependency makes a decision to turn his or her life over to the care of God. If that's too big a step for the individual, then he or she turns life over to the care of a power higher than him- or herself, which might be the group. Self-reliance gives way to reliance on God. In passing, it is worth noting that this is the object of everyone's journey in faith. It is for this very reason that the founders of the AA program called alcohol dependency a spiritual disease.

Twelve-step programs as a rule have sponsorship built into their structure. Participants are strongly encouraged (not required) to ask someone with a bit of time in the program to be their sponsor. This person listens, is available for calls, and generally keeps the other focused on working the program. Thus the possibility of being accountable to someone else is part of the way many of these self-help programs operate.

Accessibility

While certain professional resources can be scarce in some locations, self-help groups proliferate in almost every community. Although people in extremely remote parts of the country may have to drive 30 to 50 miles for a meeting, most of the time meetings are much closer. Urban areas, in fact, often offer smoking, nonsmoking, morning, lunch, and evening meetings, as well as a host of other variations for some kinds of groups.

Savvy and Resilience

Most self-help groups offer an organizational culture that equips lay people to deal with the addictive behaviors and traumatic emotions of others. While an adult church school class likely would be hard-pressed to deal with a member who arrived intoxicated, for example, an AA group would have a much clearer idea of how to help the person. Because of their experience, self-help groups are able to cope with trauma that would exhaust many other groups, whether that trauma be from a diagnosis of schizophrenia in a family member or chronic cocaine use.

Self-Help Groups and the Church

Just as self-help groups are not a substitute for professional assistance when that is what is required, so also they are not a substitute for the church. The roles of the church and the self-help group in an individual's growth can be highly complementary. The relationship, however, can be compromised from either side.

Occasionally members of self-help groups say that the church is not as effective in helping them as their groups, which is likely to be true in terms of their specific challenge. Self-help groups have a special culture that teaches persons how to deal with their particular challenge. More frequently the complaint is lodged that people do not feel as comfortable in a church as they do in their twelve-step group. Sometimes this charge is sad but true. It can be a sign of how far from the experience of koinonia—community with Christ and with one another—the church has sometimes strayed. People in a twelve-step group share their experience, strength, and hope with one another. Ideally, that description includes what people in the church do, too.

Yet the church's role is far wider. Even if someone finds specialized aid in a group that he or she can't find in church, that group is not equipped to help a person grow in his or her faith life. This is where the church serves a complementary role. Bill Wilson, one of the founders of AA, wrote, "We are only operating a spiritual kindergarten in which people are enabled to get over drinking and find the grace to go on living to better effect. Each man's theology has to be his own quest, his own affair."[6] That quest is where the church steps in.

Some people in the church are also hostile to self-help groups. This resistance may arise out of fear that the groups are in competition with the church or be based on a particular experience with a self-help group or members of one. In either case, a blanket resistance is unwarranted and unnecessarily limits people's options for finding help for a given problem. Church leaders can help by accurately communicating the purpose of self-help groups and making it possible for self-help groups to use church facilities.

Churches and self-help groups can assist each other in meeting each organization's goals. Churches can support individuals in need of a self-help group by helping persons locate a group, encouraging them in their attendance, and providing a place for groups to meet. Self-help groups help persons overcome difficulties that impede their ability to be whole persons—a need that exists among Christians, too—and by providing focused care that the church is usually unable to provide.

Self-Help Groups and Stephen Ministry

Some of a Stephen Ministry's care receivers may be involved in one or more self-help groups. In many instances there will be no conflict between being a member of a self-help group and having a Stephen Minister. Often the two resources together can multiply the emotional support that a person has for coping with his or her situation.

Sometimes, however, participation in a self-help group combined with receiving care from a Stephen Minister is not sufficient to address a care receiver's needs. Stephen Leaders and Stephen Ministers should be aware of situations such as

6 [William Wilson], *As Bill Sees It: The A.A. Way of Life* (New York: Alcoholics Anonymous World Services, Inc., 1967), p. 95.

the following, which are inappropriate as caring situations for Stephen Ministers.

- A care receiver involved in a grief support group whose mourning is turning into moderate or severe depression and who therefore needs a referral to a physician or a mental health professional for assessment

- A person with a diagnosis of schizophrenia who refuses to accept psychiatric support, joins a support group for persons with this diagnosis, and requests a Stephen Minister

A Stephen Minister could appropriately work with such persons only when they are under the care of a mental health professional and when the Stephen Minister is serving with the permission and guidance of the professional caregiver.

Whatever the situation—whether a care receiver is already part of a self-help group and wants a Stephen Minister, the care receiver wants to join a self-help group while in a Stephen Ministry relationship, or the Stephen Minister believes a self-help group would be beneficial to the care receiver and wants to make a referral—it may be helpful to seek the advice of a mental health professional. The mental health professional can assist in discerning the best type of care for a care receiver. He or she can also offer a recommendation regarding whether the Stephen Ministry relationship should continue and, if so, how the Stephen Minister can best support the care receiver. The mental health professional may also be able to offer suggestions regarding the most appropriate self-help groups in your area.

With regard to the first three types of groups, for illness, for caregivers, and for those suffering tragedies, a congregation's Stephen Ministry should also do its own research about available self-help groups. Despite their strengths, some of these self-help groups may be unhealthy or ineffective. This may vary from group to group within the same support organization. Ideally, Stephen Leaders should get information about local groups ahead of time so that when someone is in need of a self-help group, he or she can be referred quickly. If money is involved, or a group has an unsavory reputation in the community, or if there are indications that a group might try to control people's lives in a cultlike fashion, make sure that your Stephen Ministers don't refer care receivers to such a group.

Many Stephen Ministries are blessed with Stephen Leaders, Stephen Ministers, pastors, or other church staff who have had some experience in self-help groups and are willing to break their anonymity for the sake of sharing what they know. If your congregation's Stephen Ministry has such a credible information resource, rely on it.

•••

In summary, self-help groups can exist in harmony alongside professional treatment, the church, and Stephen Ministry. Keys to such harmony are asking the right questions and gaining a thorough understanding of the resources available in your area.

4

Mental Health Professionals

Stephen Ministers and mental health professionals each have a distinctive and valuable place in offering care to people in need. Many situations require the kind of compassionate presence that you can provide as a Stephen Minister. Less frequently, a person needs the more intensive, focused, and highly trained care that a mental health professional can provide. In a small number of Stephen Ministry relationships, professional care will replace or be used in addition to Stephen Ministry. That is why Stephen Leaders and Stephen Ministers need to be aware of the various types of mental health professionals and the kinds of services they provide.

Mental health professionals receive extensive specialized training and are licensed by the states in which they practice. They often have other certifications granted by various accrediting bodies within their specialties. They are held accountable by the states who license them, the institutions and organizations that employ them, and the professional associations that accredit them. They are paid for their services by the persons they help, by a third party such as an insurance company, or a combination of the two.

Types of Mental Health Professionals

Stephen Ministry congregations need to keep up-to-date information about qualified mental health professionals who can serve their members when the need arises. Ideally, this list would include professionals from more than one discipline and perhaps more than one option within a single discipline. The variety of degrees, titles, accreditations, and specialties can be confusing to someone who is not familiar with the mental health community, so this chapter contains a basic overview of the primary types of mental health professionals.

Types of Mental Health Professionals

- Clinical psychologists

- Clinical social workers

- Counseling psychologists

- Counselors

- Marriage and family counselors

- Pastoral counselors

- Psychiatric nurses

- Psychiatrists

The following categories (listed alphabetically) include some basic types of mental health professionals. While not comprehensive, it gives Stephen Leaders, pastors, and you a place to start in locating mental health professionals in your congregation's community. Be aware that titles and qualifications vary somewhat from state to state, and often more so outside the United States. There is a good deal of overlap in who treats what kinds of problems, so don't take these categories as mutually exclusive.

Clinical Psychologists

Clinical psychologists have doctor's degrees (Ph.D. or Psy.D.) in psychology. In addition to their academic course work, clinical psychologists complete an intensive regimen of patient treatment under supervision and pass a state licensing examination. These mental health professionals typically specialize in various types of psychotherapy and often use psychological tests in diagnosis.

Problems that concern a clinical psychologist range from normal psychological crises related to personal growth, such as teenage rebellion and midlife crisis, to such extreme conditions as schizophrenia or bipolar disorder. Clinical psychologists typically do not prescribe medications themselves but will usually have access to psychiatrists, who can prescribe needed medication. Many clinical psychologists work within a professional group that includes psychiatrists, social workers, and others. The American Psychological Association develops and oversees standards of practice and maintains a code of ethics for clinical psychologists.

To Stephen Leaders

As you develop your list, keep in mind that mental health professionals vary in their approach and effectiveness, even within groups with the same credentials. In some states a person can call him- or herself a counselor or therapist without any training at all. The other side of the coin is that degrees, licensure, and other certifications by themselves are not sufficient to qualify a person as a referral source. Appendix D offers suggestions on how to find a competent professional to work with care receivers who need referral.

Part of your responsibility as you select and screen mental health professionals for possible use by your congregation's Stephen Ministry is to help those individuals understand what Stephen Ministry is. Your best help here is probably this book; second best, the video called *Stephen Ministry and Mental Health Issues*. In addition, use Friends Packets—the collection of printed materials that is distributed by Stephen Ministries St. Louis—to share with the

Clinical Social Workers

Clinical social workers have master's, and sometimes doctor's, degrees in social work and have met state licensing requirements. Like other mental health professionals, they have completed extensive clinical training in their field.

mental health professionals who are willing and qualified to serve as resources for your congregation.

A licensed clinical social worker performs psychotherapy and can be especially helpful in assessing how an individual's environment affects his or her behavior. Typical areas of focus for licensed clinical social workers include the following.

- Chemical dependency

- Depression

- Marriage and family counseling

- Medical conditions; for example, counseling patients with AIDS

- Child and adolescent issues

- Inpatient psychiatric issues

- Follow-up to hospitalization

The National Association of Social Workers develops and oversees standards of practice and adherence to a code of ethics for the profession.

Counseling Psychologists

Counseling psychologists have a doctor's degree (Ph.D., Psy.D., or Ed.D.) and adhere to standards and ethics established by the American Psychological Association. Their training focuses on working with people experiencing normal psychological problems more than with those requiring hospitalization. They often do short-term treatment to help people adjust to normal developmental issues, but they also treat those with problems associated with physical, emotional, and mental disorders. Counseling psychologists also often help people with vocational concerns.

Counselors

Professional counselors have master's or doctor's degrees in counseling and, if licensed, have met state licensing requirements. Some professional counselors treat various individual and family problems, while others may specialize in areas such as eating disorders or substance abuse. Other areas of concern include helping individuals:

- make sound educational and career decisions and develop their potential;

- cope with physical and emotional crises;

- resolve personal and family conflicts such as separation, divorce, remarriage, abuse, being a stepparent, custody issues, or sexuality concerns; or

- develop life skills for dealing with transition and change.

The National Board for Certified Counselors monitors a process to certify qualified counselors. The National Academy of Certified Clinical Mental Health Counselors certifies qualified clinical mental health counselors who meet specific education, experience, and competency-based clinical skills criteria.

Marriage and Family Counselors

Marriage and family counselors have master's or doctor's degrees in counseling-related fields and have met state licensing requirements for marriage and family counseling.

A marriage and family counselor usually works with issues that involve the dynamics of relationships within a family.

Typical areas of concern for marriage and family counselors include the following.

• Child behavior problems

• Abusive relationships

• Divorce or separation

The American Association of Marriage and Family Therapists develops and oversees standards of practice and adherence to a code of ethics for these counselors and for professionals from other disciplines who focus on working with families.

Pastoral Counselors

While all pastors have some duties that can be called counseling in a broad sense, pastoral counselors have received specialized training to help people address mental, emotional, spiritual, and relational issues. Pastoral counselors may be ordained or nonordained persons, but all have a special ability to draw upon their and their clients' faith resources to bring about healing.

Pastoral counselors may be found in a variety of locations. Some work in larger clinics attached to hospitals; others may be in small group practices, work as individual therapists, or be attached to a local congregation. In some states they are licensed as pastoral counselors; elsewhere they may be licensed as clinical psychologists, social workers, or clinical professional counselors, depending on their training and degrees.

The American Association of Pastoral Counselors provides certification and oversight for this group of therapists.

Psychiatric Nurses

Psychiatric nurses are licensed registered nurses who specialize in mental health issues. A psychiatric nurse, certified, has completed additional study and training beyond his or her bachelor's degree in nursing. A psychiatric mental health clinical specialist, certified, has a master's degree in psychiatric nursing, including supervised clinical training. Such a person is also designated an Advanced Practice Nurse. State Boards of Nursing determine licensing requirements. The American Nurses Association sets national standards of practice.

Psychiatric nurses may focus on selected populations (e.g., family, children and youth, chronically mentally ill) or specific problems (e.g., emotional crisis, chemical dependency, depression). They work effectively with persons who have both medical and emotional problems.

Psychiatric nurses frequently work on a treatment team in a hospital or outpatient setting. They typically have the most direct contact with a person and that individual's family. The psychiatric mental health clinical specialist works in these settings or in private practice. This treatment role in some states includes having access to a physician, usually a psychiatrist, who will prescribe medication as needed.

Psychiatrists

Psychiatrists are medical doctors who specialize in diagnosing and treating psychiatric disorders. They work with a variety of problems, often in close liaison with other mental health professionals, but are more likely to focus on more debilitating mental disorders, such as schizophrenia. As a medical doctor, a psychiatrist can prescribe medications and admit people to hospitals for inpatient treatment.

Psychiatrists may specialize in a particular area such as

---

geriatrics, chemical addiction, or child and adolescent psychiatry, to name a few. Upon passing exams offered by the American Board of Psychiatry and Neurology, they are said to be board certified. The American Psychiatric Association is generally responsible for standards of practice issues and adherence to a code of ethics. They can verify the credentials of a particular practitioner.

For More Information

This brief survey of mental health professionals serves as a general orientation to help you understand what kinds of professionals are available to help care receivers. More information is available in books about therapies and mental health professionals and from community resource directories.

Clinics or Private Practice

The kind of mental health treatment you would seek out for your care receiver when a referral is necessary depends mainly on the particular needs of the care receiver and on the type and quality of treatment services that are available in your area.

A person who needs specialized help may see several of the professionals described in this chapter at various times during his or her treatment. For example, someone may go to a clinic and be under the care of a psychiatrist for prescription medication, a psychologist for testing, and a social worker for therapy. Because clinics usually have on their staff several professionals with various specialties who normally function as a treatment team, a care receiver may be able to get everything he or she needs in one place, whether it is medication, testing, or therapy.

When using a clinic or other type of counseling group as a resource for referrals, it is always best to know each professional to whom you might eventually refer and, if possible, refer only to those professionals whom you know and trust. In some cases, you may be able to develop a good working relationship with one professional on a clinic's staff who then refers within that center.

Of course, if you work with an agency you may not have the luxury of choice that you would when working with a mental health professional in private practice. While mental health professionals who have their own private practice are available in many communities, clinics or teams of professionals are more available in larger municipal areas. If both options are available, your congregation may want to establish relationships with both solo practitioners and clinics, for there are unique advantages to both.

> **To the Stephen Leader**
>
> In researching a clinic, note that you will probably have less ability to choose which therapist your care receiver will be assigned to. Find out how the clinic decides which mental health professional will be assigned to a client and whether the clinic understands and will honor your need for care receivers to be assigned therapists who will respect their Christian faith.

Christian or Non-Christian

When you seek professional care for your care receiver, should the mental health professional be a Christian? This is a challenging question, and there are several important factors to take into account.

Ideally, it would be best to find a highly effective mental health professional who was a committed Christian whose own belief system was compatible with the Christian beliefs of your care receiver. But that may not always be possible, in which case your primary consideration needs to be whether the mental health professional is effective. The essential requirement is that the individual you select for referral is a competent, effective mental health professional who respects the care receiver's faith and affirms its importance to the care receiver. He or she must accept the role that Christian faith plays in the care receiver's life. If the professional does not have the ability to discuss faith issues effectively, he or she can encourage the client to seek spiritual help from clergy or other Christians.

There may even be times when selecting a Christian mental health professional could create more problems for the care receiver. Some Christian therapists may have theological views that could conflict with your own tradition or denomination. If these professionals regularly share or teach their own theological views that disagree with a care receiver's beliefs, they may confuse a care receiver. Stephen Leaders and the church staff need to use discernment in finding qualified Christian therapists and in avoiding those who, for various reasons, would not serve the needs of members of your congregation.

Some professionals advertise that they are Christian psychiatrists, psychologists, or counselors, sometimes by putting a fish or a cross in a Yellow Pages advertisement or on a business card. Should you look for mental health professionals who advertise themselves in that way? Possibly. Yet a Christian label by itself does not guarantee either professional competence or sound Christian theology.

On the other hand, there are many competent mental health professionals who do not advertise that they are Christian yet are no less serious about matters of faith. These Christians manage their practices as people of faith and provide high-quality care without publicizing their religious affiliation. They talk about their Christian beliefs when it is fitting to do so within a given therapeutic relationship. It is possible, therefore, to find competent, committed Christian mental health professionals among those who do not advertise their services as Christian.

It is certainly appropriate for Christians in mental health professions to describe themselves as Christian therapists. Appendix D will help your Stephen Ministry evaluate mental health professionals and find ones who are competent and who will respect the faith of care receivers your congregation refers to them.

Mental Health Professionals Serving as Stephen Ministers

Having mental health professionals volunteer to go through training to be Stephen Ministers is no different than having hairdressers, lawyers, or plumbers volunteer. A Stephen Minister who happens also to be a mental health professional needs to be aware of two possible pitfalls, however: giving care that is not appropriate for a Stephen Minister to give, or inappropriately benefiting by his or her role (for example, using it to get more clients).

The following suggestions can help mental health professionals serve ethically and effectively as a Stephen Minister.

For Mental Health Professionals Serving as Stephen Leaders

Many mental health professionals serve very successfully as Stephen Leaders. Here are some guidelines for such ministry.

1. Work within the Stephen Series system in the same way any other Stephen Leader would. Your mental health background should not cause you to implement Stephen Ministry in your congregation differently than any non-mental health professional Stephen Leader would. Mental health professionals should stick to the basic Stephen Series system just as a Stephen

1. Since you will be a Stephen Minister, do what Stephen Ministers normally do. Be ready to refer if it becomes apparent that your care receiver needs a mental health professional.

2. Downplay your profession, particularly in relationship to your care receiver. If your care receiver asks what you do for a living, say something like, "I work as a _____, but of course I don't do that with you. Here I'm your Stephen Minister."

3. Do not allow yourself to be connected with a care receiver who needs professional counseling. If you believe a care receiver needs a mental health professional's help, decline the ministry assignment and explain why you are doing so. Occasionally there will be a tricky caregiving situation in which a Stephen Minister with a high level of maturity or life experience may be needed. If it is your maturity as a Stephen Minister and as a person that motivates the Stephen Leaders' assigning you, and not the fact that

Leader who is a banker or hairdresser would.

2. Resist the temptation to include material or information inappropriate for lay caregivers in continuing education. Material dealing with issues beyond the scope of lay ministry—dream analysis, for example—should not become part of Stephen Ministry training at any level.

3. Make caregiving assignments based strictly on the criteria found in the Stephen Ministry resources. For example, be wary of thinking that, since you will be the Supervision Group Facilitator for a particular Stephen Minister's Supervision Group, she or he can be placed in a caregiving situation beyond the capabilities of a lay caregiver.

4. When mental health issues arise in caregiving situations, include other mental health professionals as outside consultants in making decisions about treatment. They can provide an extra

you are a mental health professional, then by all means accept the assignment.

4. If during the course of a caregiving relationship as a Stephen Minister you come to realize that your care receiver needs a mental health professional, this person should not be referred to you but to another mental health professional.

5. Do not bring into supervision any information you might have learned about a care receiver through your work as a mental health professional.

The reasons for these guidelines are self-evident in terms of ethical and liability issues. This is similar to the distinction other professionals must make. For instance, a lawyer who serves as a Stephen Minister would blur the caring relationship if he or she gave legal counsel to the care receiver; so would a physician who is a Stephen Minister who gave medical treatment.

degree of objectivity and often can offer you a fresh perspective. Along this same line, do not accept referrals to your personal practice from your congregation's Stephen Ministry. Your professional knowledge and experience can be valuable assets to your Stephen Ministry in other ways: for example, in helping determine the specific criteria and questions your Stephen Leader Team will use to evaluate another professional as a potential consultant to your Stephen Ministry.

The bottom line is this:

Keep the boundaries clear between your occupation as a mental health professional and your service as a Stephen Leader.

Blurring the distinctions between Stephen Ministry and mental health practice also can undermine the effectiveness of a congregation's Stephen Ministry. A Stephen Leader or Stephen Minister in the mental health field who acts as an "expert" can intimidate other members of the

Stephen Ministry. They may feel inadequate in their skills and defer to the mental health professional. Supervision could shift away from the peer emphasis and become a meeting where a group of laypeople sit at the feet of an expert. Bringing too much of your knowledge and training into Stephen Ministry can also wrongly influence the congregation's expectations of what its Stephen Ministry can provide. People may come to expect professionally qualified care rather than distinctively Christian lay caregiving ministry.

The relationship between the caregiver and the care receiver in each role is also different. A mental health professional typically has no outside relationship with his or her clients. As a Stephen Minister, however, you would have contact with some of the care receivers through the congregation's normal functions. For these reasons and others, being both a mental health professional and a Stephen Minister can be challenging. Despite these challenges, many mental health professionals find serving as a Stephen Minister very rewarding.

One psychiatrist gave a hint of these rewards. He retired from his position in his state's mental health system, then trained to be a Stephen Minister. He said, "I used to be able only to pray for my patients, but now I can pray with my care receivers."

If you are a mental health professional serving as a Stephen Minister, check with your congregation's insurance carrier or a lawyer to be clear about any legal liability connected with your functioning in that role. Does the carrier see your role as a mental health professional and your role as a lay caregiver as being separate and distinct? What does a lawyer have to say about potential liability problems?

You should also check with your own insurance carrier, describe what you will be doing as a Stephen Minister, and see if your insurance provider has any problems with your participating in that ministry.

Identify whatever risk there may be both for your congregation and for you and do what is necessary to minimize that risk.

• • •

Mental health professionals are an essential adjunct to your congregation's providing appropriate care to those in need. Knowing about mental health professionals is the first step toward working well with them, and this chapter has addressed that first step. Subsequent chapters will include how to get to know some mental health professionals so that you can confidently recommend them to people who need their care.

5

When to Refer a Care Receiver to a Mental Health Resource

Suzanne had been Donna's Stephen Minister for three months following the death of Donna's husband, Roger, who had a six-month bout with cancer. Roger's death had been very hard on Donna, especially since she and Roger were just beginning to enjoy their empty nest after their youngest child moved out of the state.

About two weeks after the funeral, Donna went back to work. Donna loved her work very much and believed it would be good to begin resuming her normal routine. Suzanne supported her in that choice.

During a visit a month ago, Donna mentioned to Suzanne that she had missed work the day before because she had felt too tired to go. Given her recent loss, her employer had been very understanding and supportive of Donna. The following week Donna told Suzanne that she had missed two days of work. Suzanne mentioned this to her Supervision Group. The members advised Suzanne to be on the lookout for future occurrences. Donna was still obviously grieving, but she did appear to be keeping up with her other life obligations.

At their meeting today, however, Donna told Suzanne that she had missed work twice more in the past week, again because she felt tired. Suzanne also noticed that Donna's usually immaculate home was beginning to look more cluttered. In addition, Donna, who typically was very stylish, was looking a bit disheveled and was not wearing any makeup. She appeared slightly distracted to Suzanne. Donna insisted, however, that she was fine and would be going to work the next day. Suzanne knew she needed to discuss what she had observed with her Supervision Group, which was meeting the next evening. She called her Supervision Group Facilitator after her visit with Donna to say she needed to give an in-depth report at tomorrow night's Supervision Group, even though it was not her turn.

Sometimes care receivers find problems to be so intense and difficult to deal with that their needs go beyond the scope of a Stephen Minister's skills and training. For this reason, mental health professionals are essential partners in any congregation's overall caregiving. They exist alongside the caregiving ministries of the congregation. This chapter describes some of the situations in which referrals to mental health professionals are necessary, or at least should be explored in consultation.

When to Consider Referral

Referrals of care receivers to mental health professionals should be made in order to:

- provide appropriate care for care receivers who need help from a professional caregiver; and

- strengthen Stephen Ministry by freeing Stephen Ministers to do what they have been trained to do or by giving them additional support in dealing with difficult caregiving situations.

There are three critical occasions in Stephen Ministry to consider referral to a mental health professional: during the preparation interview, when the care receiver's needs become clearer, and when changes occur during a caring relationship.

During the Preparation Interview

When Stephen Leaders first find out about a possible care receiver, the Referrals Coordinator (or another Stephen Leader) conducts a preparation interview. It is in the course of this interview that the Stephen Leader assesses whether Stephen Ministry is appropriate for this care receiver.

It may be easy to see during this interview that the care receiver needs professional care. If a care receiver is asking for someone to minister to him or her and his or her spouse to improve their marriage, for example, the choice is clear. Stephen Ministers do not work conjointly with care receivers, and they are not qualified to help solve relational difficulties. Other examples of referrals that are clearly unsuitable for Stephen Ministers include care receivers suffering from severe depression or addiction who are not already under a professional's care. (See chapter 2, pages 37–47, for more about what Stephen Ministers do not do.)

In other instances, however, it will not be so easy to decide whether the care receiver needs professional care or Stephen Ministry. If a care receiver is depressed, it may be difficult for the Referrals Coordinator to assess whether the depression is mild, moderate, or severe. If the Referrals Coordinator has doubts about assigning a care receiver to a Stephen Minister, he or she needs to take those doubts seri-

---

To Stephen Leaders

The reference to depression here serves to highlight the importance of having all Stephen Leaders learn what Stephen Ministers learn in their training. Guidelines to follow in determining whether someone is depressed enough to warrant professional care are taught in the Stephen Ministry training module

---

ously, as does a Stephen Minister who has doubts about continuing with a care receiver. In such cases the Referrals Coordinator should consult with a trusted mental health professional and then follow that advice.

When the Care Receiver's Needs Become Clearer

"Dealing with Depression: The Stephen Minister's Role." This is only one reason why effective Stephen Leaders will seek to master the content of Stephen Minister training, either by teaching it or by attending the sessions that other Stephen Leaders teach.

A care receiver also may be referred to a mental health professional when his or her needs become clearer than they originally were. The care receiver may have needed professional help all along, but the Referrals Coordinator or other Stephen Leader did not detect the need at the time of the preparation interview. Even highly trained mental health professionals sometimes need more than one interview to fully understand a client's needs. Some persons experiencing serious emotional problems may intentionally or unintentionally mask what is really going on with them. As the Stephen Ministry relationship develops, however, it may become clear that this care receiver is unable to deal with his or her challenges and that he or she needs more help than a Stephen Minister can give.

The care receiver's need may become clearer as he or she shares new information about his or her condition with you. For example, after a number of caring visits a care receiver might reveal that he or she has been abusing alcohol or some other drug.

When Changes Occur during a Caring Relationship

A care receiver who was appropriate for a Stephen Minister can undergo changes that take his or her needs beyond those a Stephen Minister is qualified to care for.

Changes That Signal a Referral to a Mental Health Professional

If any of these changes occur, talk to your Stephen Leader or Supervision Group about making a referral to a mental health professional.

- *The care receiver's situation gets worse,* such as when a grieving care receiver who is mildly depressed slips into a severe depression.

- *The nature of the care receiver's problem changes,* as, for example, when a person who has needed crisis and follow-up care during a divorce starts hearing voices telling him to get back together with his wife.

Whenever you suspect that your care receiver's needs may have changed and that he or she now requires professional care, you should act quickly. Even if you aren't sure the care receiver needs professional care, you need to talk to your Supervision Group or Stephen Leaders to get help with beginning to assess the situation.

Making the Decision to Refer

Regardless of when the need for a referral becomes evident, making the decision to refer a care receiver to a mental health professional can prove challenging. But it isn't a decision you need to make alone.

Resistance to Deciding to Refer

Stephen Ministers may resist deciding to make a referral to a mental health professional for several reasons. They may be enjoying the caring relationship and worry that a referral will mean they have to end it. A Stephen Minister may also believe that he or she can handle the care receiver's situation, or ought to be able to handle it, and think that making a referral means admitting failure. Stephen Ministers may also be afraid of what their peers will think of them if they refer their care receiver.

Care receivers also may resist a decision to refer them to a mental health professional for a number of reasons, but you will learn ways to deal with this resistance in the next chapter, on pages 110–114.

A Shared Decision

Fortunately, you do not have to decide about referrals on your own. The decision to refer a care receiver to a mental health professional needs to be one that you share with your Supervision Group, Stephen Leaders, or pastor.

If you suspect that a care receiver needs professional care, bring that possibility up with your Supervision Group. Even if you are not scheduled to discuss your caring relationship in depth, you should consider this a need to go to the front of the line for help from the Supervision Group. The Supervision Group can use "Focus Question Set H: Focus on a Possible Mental Health Referral" (see appendix A, pages 141–142) to help you decide what to do next in the caring relationship.

If you believe that the care receiver might be in imminent danger of committing suicide or harming others, you must do whatever it takes to ensure the safety of persons. Generally that means contacting a Stephen Leader, pastor, mental health professional, the police, or some other authority immediately. If contacting a Stephen Leader or pastor would delay getting help for the care receiver, however, you should dial 911 or otherwise contact the police immediately.

In an emergency involving suicide, homicide, or abuse, you do not even need the care receiver's permission to get help. The need to preserve a life outweighs your commitment to confidentiality.[1]

Key Questions for Determining Whether a Referral to a Mental Health Professional Is in Order

Note that the "Agreement to Receive Care" in appendix E, which your Referrals Coordinator may have had the care receiver sign before your caring relationship began, already paves the way for a referral to a professional should the necessity arise. The following list of questions will help your Referrals Coordinator and you to assess whether a care receiver needs a mental health professional's care. Supervision Group Facilitators and Supervision Group members should also keep these questions in mind as they help you determine whether a referral is needed. If the answer is yes to any of these questions, it's time to consider seriously referral to a mental health professional.

Questions to Use in Assessing Whether a Care Receiver Needs a Mental Health Professional

- Does the person seem to be having difficulty maintaining the basic functions of life?

- Has the person experienced marked weight loss or gain?

- Would you expect the care receiver to be doing significantly better by now?

- Does the care receiver's ability to cope seem to be on a definite downward spiral?

- Is the care receiver becoming overly dependent on the Stephen Minister?

1 For more information on the three exceptions to confidentiality, review the Stephen Minister training module 9, "Confidentiality," in your *Stephen Ministry Training Manual*.

- Has the person become extremely withdrawn from his or her usual social activities?

- Is the person involved in any kind of abusive situation?

- Is the care receiver behaving explosively or threatening violence?

- Does the person seem disoriented or out of touch with reality? For example, is there any evidence of auditory or visual hallucinations?

- Has the person mentioned suicidal thoughts or wishes or behaved in reckless, self-destructive ways?

Does the Person Seem to Be Having Difficulty Maintaining the Basic Functions of Life?

Inability to cope could be indicated by any of the following signs.

- Absence from work

- Inability to attend church

- Inability to maintain one's living environment or personal hygiene

- Mismanagement of finances

- Inappropriate expression of feelings

- Overreaction to typical life challenges

- Increased conflict with one's spouse, family, or friends

The psychological term for this is *decompensation*. Areas of a person's life that were under control start to fall apart as the struggle with emotional pain demands more attention.

Has the Person Experienced Marked Weight Loss or Gain?

Marked weight loss or gain can have physical causes or can be associated with emotional and mental problems. The first referral in such instances, therefore, might be to the care receiver's physician.

Would You Expect the Care Receiver to Be Doing Significantly Better by Now?

Consider whether the care receiver seems to be stuck in one spot, based on what you observe during visits, but also on what seems to be occurring in the rest of the care receiver's life. For example, if a care receiver has suffered a major loss, it is normal to go through a time of denial in which he or she doesn't admit to the reality or the meaning of the loss and doesn't show grief feelings. If a care receiver gets stuck in such denial, however, that is not healthy and the person probably needs professional help. Granger Westberg says: "This shock stage—or perhaps it should be called a counter shock—may last anywhere from a few minutes to a few hours to a few days. If it goes on for some weeks, it probably is unhealthy grief and professional help ought to be sought."[2] Be sure to consider all aspects of the situation carefully, however, remembering that it can take a long time to work through a crisis, grief, loss, or other painful circumstance.

Does the Care Receiver's Ability to Cope Seem to Be on a Definite Downward Spiral?

A definite downward spiral may be evident in a number of areas and may be the result of new crises or of changes in a person's circumstances. For example, a care receiver had been assigned to a Stephen Minister because she felt alone and suffered low self-esteem. Then her boss yelled at her

---

2 Granger E. Westberg, *Good Grief: A Constructive Approach to the Problem of Loss* (Philadelphia: Fortress Press, 1971), p. 21.

and put her on probation, which filled her with dread that she was going to be fired. When her boyfriend broke up with her, she stopped going to work. Finally, the care receiver threatened suicide and refused all efforts to get professional help until the Stephen Minister let her know that there was no alternative.

Additional traumas in any care receiver's life may make it more difficult to cope with the original situation. Physical illness in addition to an emotional problem, for example, can greatly decrease a care receiver's ability to cope.

A care receiver's reactions to existing circumstances can also change. There is no new trauma, but the care receiver decompensates, meaning his or her ability to cope with what was already going on deteriorates.

Is the Care Receiver Becoming Overly Dependent on the Stephen Minister?

Overdependence can be indicated by excessive reliance on the Stephen Minister. The care receiver may begin calling the Stephen Minister every day for help with the simplest decisions and refuse to take responsibility for him- or herself. This could indicate that the person is becoming unable to function adequately on his or her own. If a care receiver is constantly challenging appropriate boundaries in the relationship, then probably a mental health professional is the right one to be working with the care receiver.

Has the Person Become Extremely Withdrawn from His or Her Usual Social Activities?

A care receiver who becomes withdrawn and distant may be signaling the need for referral to a mental health professional. This is true especially if such behavior is quite different from the person's normal demeanor and practice. For instance, if a person has always been one of the "regulars" and then stops attending events at church or in the community, this could be evidence of the need for a professional evaluation.

Is the Person Involved in Any Kind of Abusive Situation?

Victims of abuse can include elders, spouses, and children. Abuse can be physical, emotional, sexual, or combinations of these. It can even include such violence as assault or rape. If you learn of abuse that is going on, whether the care receiver is the abuser or the abused person, you must take whatever other mandatory steps your locality requires. Your Stephen Leaders will have done the research already to determine your locality's reporting requirements and the

To the Stephen Leader

Note well your need to have done this research about mandatory local reporting requirements before you assign care receivers to your Stephen Ministers. Since laws, procedures, and agencies change, periodically verify that your research is current.

possible ramifications of making a report. Your Stephen Leader should also have on hand the telephone numbers of area shelters in case of an emergency. Whatever the law may or may not require, your concern is based on Christian love and you are going to do your best to make sure the person gets the help he or she needs, which may include referral to a mental health professional.

Is the Care Receiver Behaving Explosively or Threatening Violence?

Violent behavior or threats, to the caregiver or others, are danger signs to take seriously in all cases. If you believe there is an immediate danger of violence, you need to do what is necessary to assure your own safety and then call the police. Remember that homicidal behavior is one of the instances in which you must suspend confidentiality and take action immediately.

If you don't think there is an immediate threat, you need to consult as soon as possible with a Stephen Leader and a mental health professional to decide what step to take next.

Does the Person Seem Disoriented or Out of Touch with Reality?

Is the person's speech inconsistent and incoherent? Does the person seem to be having auditory or visual hallucinations: hearing or seeing something that you don't hear or see? Are there other evidences of radical personality changes or delusions? Is the care receiver engaging in any unusual behavior? Does the care receiver report that he or she has stopped, or is going to stop, taking essential medication? In instances where the ability to function either emotionally or physically is aided by medications, not taking them can lead to setbacks and, in some cases, be life-threatening.

Has the Person Mentioned Suicidal Thoughts or Wishes or Behaved in Reckless, Self-Destructive Ways?

Review the material in chapter 2 (pages 45–46) about assessing suicide risk. This material also refers you to the Stephen Minister training module on "Helping Suicidal Persons Get the Help They Need."

Seven Bad Reasons for Not Referring to a Mental Health Professional

Sometimes people can talk themselves into going against their better judgment. No one is exempt from this tendency.

It can show up when a Referrals Coordinator knows that a care receiver really needs professional help but assigns a Stephen Minister instead. It could show itself when you think your care receiver may need a referral to a mental health professional but you do not share that thought with your Supervision Group. The following seven statements vividly illustrate some of the ways that Stephen Leaders could talk themselves into making inappropriate referrals or you can talk yourself into continuing a Stephen Ministry relationship past the point where it is wise to do so.

Seven Bad Reasons for Not Referring to a Mental Health Professional

1. "Since the potential care receiver cannot afford professional care, a Stephen Minister is better than nothing."

2. "The potential care receiver does not want a referral to a mental health professional. He or she wants a Stephen Minister."

3. "We have a Stephen Minister who really needs a care receiver."

4. "It would not be Christian to withhold a Stephen Minister from this person."

5. "It would not be Christian to remove the Stephen Minister from this caring relationship."

6. "We will embarrass the care receiver if we say that professional care might be needed."

7. "If we recommend professional help, the care receiver might become angry and leave the church."

---

1. *"Since the Potential Care Receiver Cannot Afford Professional Care, a Stephen Minister Would Be Better Than Nothing."*

Stephen Ministers should never be assigned, nor should they continue as the sole caregiver, out of an idea that they are "better than nothing." Stephen Ministers are never an acceptable cheap substitute for professional care when such care is needed.

Additionally, the premise that a care receiver cannot afford professional care requires careful scrutiny. It may be based more on a lack of knowledge about what the person's insurance will pay or what affordable resources are actually available.

It is true that some care receivers cannot afford professional care, but even where that is the case, it still is not a justifiable reason to assign a Stephen Minister to a care receiver who really needs a referral to a mental health professional. This can be harmful to both the caregiver and the care receiver.

A few care receivers will also use cost as an excuse for not seeking appropriate help even though they actually can afford it. If the care receiver truly cannot afford care or is simply using that as an excuse for not seeking care, someone on the church staff should work with the person to obtain the necessary professional care. This should not be the job of a Stephen Minister.

2. *"The Potential Care Receiver Does Not Want a Referral to a Mental Health Professional. He or She Wants a Stephen Minister."*

When a care receiver wants a Stephen Minister's care instead of professional care, recognize the difference between what a person may want and what the person needs. It is difficult, especially in a voluntary setting such as the church, to say no to what someone wants. Yet Stephen Leaders must be prepared to do this when a care receiver demands a Stephen Minister but really needs care from a mental health professional. You may also have to assertively state that you can't continue as a person's Stephen Minister if he or she doesn't obtain needed professional care. Of course, no one in the congregation can force a person to accept a referral to a professional, but, likewise, a care receiver should never receive a Stephen Minister or have an existing Stephen Ministry relationship continue when that form of care is unwise.

3. "We Have a Stephen Minister Who Really Needs a Care Receiver."

It can be tempting to make an inappropriate referral in order to provide every Stephen Minister with a care receiver. With this temptation, as with the previous one, recognize the difference between a want and a need. A Stephen Minister may want any care receiver he or she can get, but what he or she needs is an appropriate care receiver. It is far better to have a Stephen Minister unassigned than to risk assigning a Stephen Minister to someone who should be seeing a mental health professional. Making such a referral can cause harm to the care receiver, the Stephen Minister, and the congregation's Stephen Ministry. This may require some patience on the Stephen Minister's part, but getting an appropriate care receiver is well worth the wait.

4. "It Would Not Be Christian to Withhold a Stephen Minister from This Person."

Someone might ask, "Would Jesus refuse this person a Stephen Minister?" The answer would, of course, be yes if the person needed another kind of care. More than once church leaders have allowed misplaced guilt to cause them to take unwise actions. It is difficult to explain to a person in pain that he or she cannot have a Stephen Minister. It is, however, far easier than explaining later, perhaps after major problems, why a Stephen Minister was assigned to a situation that obviously was beyond the scope of care a Stephen Minister is trained to provide. The caring and Christian response is to encourage the care receiver to seek the type of care that is best suited to the situation he or she is facing.

5. "It Would Not Be Christian to Remove the Stephen Minister from This Caring Relationship."

It is possible to make a referral to a care receiver who initially appeared to be an appropriate candidate for Stephen Ministry care but then later turned out to need professional attention. This can happen in any congregation's Stephen Ministry. The Christian thing to do is to provide the best care for a care receiver. If you discover that a care receiver needs professional care, then you need to do your best to see that he or she receives it.

When you refer a care receiver to a mental health professional, you also may continue to provide care, with the mental health professional's permission, or your Stephen Ministry relationship may be brought to a close. Care receivers must get the care they need, and you should not feel obliged to struggle with situations that are beyond your capabilities.

6. "We Will Embarrass the Care Receiver If We Say That Professional Care Might Be Needed."

A Stephen Minister or Stephen Leader may fear that the mention of referral will cause the care receiver to feel rejected or demeaned by the very persons committed to helping him or her. It is possible, however, to approach making a referral in a very positive, nurturing fashion, as chapter 6 describes, which promotes the well-being of the care receiver and maintains his or her dignity. Fear of embarrassment must be weighed against what could happen should a care receiver not get the right kind of help. Using the "Agreement to Receive Care" (appendix E) will help defuse this situation in advance.

7. "If We Recommend Professional Help, the Care Receiver Might Become Angry and Leave the Church."

Such thinking often has as a footnote, ". . . and that family gives a lot of money every year!" Some people make staying in any relationship, even their relationship with the church, contingent on getting what they want. They may have a habit of holding the church hostage in order to get their way.

In such a case, it can be tempting for a Stephen Leader to give in and ask a Stephen Minister to start or continue in a relationship that is not suited for Stephen Ministry. Though that may seem the easy path to follow, walking on that path places the church's Stephen Ministry and its ministry in general in grave danger. It will be much harder to pick up the pieces after the decision fails than it would have been to make the right decision in the first place. Even losing a family from a congregation is not nearly as high a price to pay as damaging a congregation's entire Stephen Ministry and placing many caring relationships at risk. But since you will be referring winsomely, assertively, and lovingly—as the next chapter makes clear—you will generally not face the prospect of losing a family from the church.

• • •

You can refer a care receiver to a mental health professional when it best serves the care receiver. When that is the case, it is the right thing to do, for it also protects the Stephen Minister and the integrity of your Stephen Ministry, builds up the church, and glorifies Christ.

6

How to Refer a Care Receiver to a Mental Health Resource

Suzanne was glad that her Supervision Group was meeting that evening because she was getting more concerned about her care receiver, Donna. She had called Donna that day just to check in. Donna had gone to work, but the sound of her voice was flat and lethargic.

When her turn came to make an in-depth presentation to her Supervision Group, Suzanne shared what she had observed about Donna. She asked the group for some help in determining whether Donna needed to be referred to a mental health professional. The group used the questions in "Focus Question Set H: Focus on a Possible Mental Health Referral" (see appendix A) to aid them in their discussion. After working through several Focus Questions, they decided that Donna should be referred to a mental health professional. The group concluded that Suzanne and Bill (Suzanne's Supervision Group Facilitator) should talk with Barbara (who was the Stephen Leader serving as the Supervision Coordinator) later that evening.

At that meeting Suzanne and Bill told Barbara the important facts of the situation. Barbara also believed that the situation warranted professional care. Barbara said, "Suzanne, you and I will start the procedure together tomorrow morning by calling Dr. Moore, the clinical psychologist who has been serving as a consultant for our congregation's Stephen Ministry."

Bill said, "Suzanne, are you going to be comfortable with pursuing this referral? I know you've never faced an issue like this as a Stephen Minister."

"Thanks, Bill," Suzanne said. "I appreciate your concern. I think I'm okay with it."

Barbara and Bill reassured Suzanne of their support for her and promised to help her as she proceeded. The three of them prayed together and agreed that they would meet again before Suzanne discussed the situation with her care receiver.

Suzanne and Barbara called Dr. Moore the next morning and told him the symptoms of depression that Suzanne had observed in Donna. Based on what he heard, Dr. Moore believed that a referral was definitely the proper way to care for Donna. He offered Suzanne several tips for presenting the idea to Donna. "I wouldn't wait on this," he said. "Contact her as soon as possible."

Suzanne and Barbara then went to the congregation's Community Resources Handbook *that the Stephen Leaders and Stephen Ministers had compiled. They studied the section that listed competent mental health professionals in the area, selected three that seemed most appropriate for Donna, and wrote down their fees, hours, locations, and other necessary information. They met again with Bill that evening, and the three of them role-played how Suzanne might present the idea of a referral to her care receiver. Suzanne then felt as prepared as she could be for discussing a mental health referral with Donna the next day.*

Referring a care receiver or potential care receiver to a mental health professional can be a very positive experience.

The purpose of the referral is to help the person receive the type of care that is best for him or her. If you confidently and clearly communicate your genuine concern for the care receiver when you suggest the referral, he or she will very likely sense it and feel good about the prospect of receiving appropriate care. Realize too that your care receiver may even be consciously or unconsciously hoping that you will suggest professional help. Many people are relieved when someone encourages them to take this step.

Steps in Making a Referral

This chapter outlines 11 steps to take in making a referral to a mental health professional.

Eleven Steps in Making a Referral

1. Watch for signs indicating the need for a referral.

2. Bring your concerns to your Supervision Group.

3. Consult with a mental health professional as necessary.

4. List some referral choices for your care receiver.

5. Decide who will talk with the care receiver.

6. Talk with the care receiver.

7. Help the care receiver make the contact.

8. Deal with the care receiver's refusal, if necessary.

9. Follow up.

10. Follow the mental health professional's directions about whether Stephen Ministry continues.

11. Continue to provide the congregation's care.

Because the rest of this chapter describes these 11 steps in great detail, this process may seem more involved than it actually is. Each step logically leads to the next, however, and taken together they are an exercise in informed common sense.

> **To the Stephen Leader Serving as Referrals Coordinator**
>
> With suitable adaptations, the 11 steps that follow can work for you too at the stage where you are initially considering whether a care receiver is an appropriate Stephen Ministry assignment.

1. Watch for Signs Indicating the Need for a Referral

You and your Stephen Leaders must be familiar with signs of a possible need for referral to a mental health professional, and you must always be watching for those indications in each care receiver. For example, you will be looking for signs that your care receiver is not making expected progress, is depending on you too much, or is unable to cope with the responsibilities of daily living. These are red flags for possible referral. Review chapter 5 for the indicators that were listed there, pages 87–92. When any of these flags go up, you need to bring your concerns to supervision.

2. Bring Your Concerns to Your Supervision Group

If possible, share your concerns with your Supervision Group before recommending a referral to your care receiver. You want to get their input about the best course of action for this particular situation.

As in the example at the beginning of this chapter, a meeting following supervision with you, your Supervision Group Facilitator, and the Supervision Coordinator is also appropriate. The Supervision Coordinator needs to know about the referral and to have a chance to offer input. The three of you can review the steps involved, develop the specific plan to follow, and determine who will take responsibility for each step. You could even role-play how you will discuss this with your care receiver. (As in the example at the beginning of this chapter, this may involve two meetings depending on the number of steps that need to be accomplished, the necessity of using an outside consultant, and other variables.)

There are times when you should seek individual supervision apart from your Supervision Group. For example, you might meet with your care receiver the day after your Supervision Group meets and note then the signs of a deepening depression. You would not wait until the next Supervision Group meeting in two weeks to discuss this. You need to call a Stephen Leader or the pastor right away to receive more timely guidance.

3. Consult with a Mental Health Professional as Necessary

In many instances, the need for referral will be straightforward. Other situations may not be clear. In these latter cases, your Stephen Leaders will probably need to assist you in contacting the mental health professional to help sort things out.

The mental health professional may recommend a referral or suggest that the situation be observed a little while longer.

To Stephen Leaders

There are three other points to keep in mind:

If you use the "Agreement to Receive Care" (appendix E), you will already have the care receiver's permission to contact a mental health professional for consultation.

A mental health professional who provides consultation on a particular Stephen Ministry relationship should not provide care to that care receiver unless this is unavoidable.

If a referral is indicated, the mental health professional can offer guidance regarding the kind of professional care that would be most appropriate for the care receiver. He or she may also give suggestions regarding the best way to approach this particular care receiver about a referral.

4. List Some Referral Choices for Your Care Receiver

With the help of the Supervision Group, Stephen Leaders, and pastor(s), compile a list of three or four mental health professionals who accept this type of referral. Make sure these professionals have already been researched and contacted by Find at least two mental health professionals to have on retainer, as you might have a lawyer for your congregation, whom you can consult whenever you have the need. Explain Stephen Ministry to them and learn enough about them that you are comfortable trusting their advice. Come to an agreement where they will be available for you to call whenever you need consultation. Agree on what you will pay them for these services. Have at least two such mental health professional consultants because one might be out of town or otherwise unavailable when you urgently need consultation.

one of your Stephen Leaders and that they have agreed to accept referrals from your congregation's Stephen Ministry. Include on the list any information you have about them, including fees, hours, specialty areas, approach to therapy, and location. (The "Mental Health Resource Information Form" in appendix D and the accompanying explanation list a number of questions to ask and provide a place to collect and store this information.)

5. Decide Who Will Talk with the Care Receiver

You, the Stephen Minister, are probably the best person to speak to the care receiver about the possibility of referral. Your relationship and the trust the two of you have developed may help the care receiver say yes. If a Stephen Leader or a member of the church staff were the first to suggest referral, the care receiver might be concerned that you had broken confidentiality. It also could lead a care receiver to think, "I really must be in bad shape; the pastor is talking to me about this." Either of those reactions may cause the care receiver to become overly anxious or to resist the idea of referral.

In some instances the pastor or another member of the church staff may be the best person to talk with the care receiver about referral. This is especially true if the pastor or staff person has a relationship with the care receiver and is familiar with his or her situation. The care receiver may also regard this person as an authority figure and value his or her recommendation. Again, tell your care receiver in advance that you need to discuss the situation confidentially with this person.

6. Talk with the Care Receiver

Following are some practical suggestions for talking with the care receiver about a mental health referral.

Pray for God's guidance and help. As always with your Stephen Ministry, you are not alone. God is right there with you helping you and bringing healing to your care receiver. Remember Paul's advice: "Let each of you look not to your own interests, but to the interests of others" (Philippians 2:4 NRSV).

Think ahead about what to say and how to say it naturally. Develop a clear and reasoned case for why a referral is appropriate. Be sure you are confident it is the right thing to do. Become comfortable with a way to phrase the idea. If possible, role-play the conversation in the Supervision Group or with an experienced Stephen Minister, Stephen

Leader, or a member of the church staff. When speaking with the care receiver, take care to avoid sounding as if you have memorized a speech. The suggestion for referral needs to come naturally and sincerely because you believe it is the right thing to do and you have the care receiver's best interests at heart.

Talk about a mental health referral as you would any other type of referral. Offer a recommendation for a mental health referral in the same way you would a physician, an attorney, or a carpenter if you noticed a board was loose on the care receiver's front steps. Try to adopt that same tone and demeanor, and keep any anxiety to a minimum. This is not to say, "Just be a good actor." Rather, your recommendation will be natural and honest because you believe that the care offered by mental health professionals is exactly what your care receiver needs.

Avoid using emotionally charged or difficult-to-understand terms or jargon. Use words or phrases that describe the care receiver's behaviors and feelings. Avoid terms that make judgments or evaluations. Instead, use some of the same words the individual has used to describe his or her situation or that you have used previously to describe the care receiver's situation. Here are examples of words and phrases that a care receiver might use and that you might repeat.

- You've said you can't concentrate on anything for more than ten seconds.

- You've said everyone and everything seem to rub you the wrong way.

- You've said you feel as if you're being crushed to bits.

- You've said you don't think you can keep going.

- You've said you are as jumpy as a cat on a hot stove.

Hearing back familiar words is an effective way to help the care receiver understand more fully, feel less threatened, and be more likely to follow through on seeking professional help.

Explain why the care receiver needs additional care. As the opportunity arises, mention that you are not a trained counselor, and therefore you cannot provide the kind of help that could bring about the needed changes in that person's life or situation. (If you happen to be a trained counselor, explain that as a Stephen Minister you are not functioning in this way.) Explain that it would be very irresponsible for you to continue to serve as the sole caregiver knowing that another kind of caregiver is really needed.

Express strong concern for the care receiver. Let the care receiver know that the suggestion for referral comes from a heartfelt concern. The care receiver needs to know that you sense his or her struggle and want to do whatever is possible to help the situation improve.

Provide a realistic message of hope. Offer a vision of a brighter future—one that is realistic, but brighter nonetheless. Speak positively about the benefits that can be attained with the right kind of help.

Be prepared for a question like, "Will it do any good?" A possible answer could be, "I do know that other people with similar problems have really benefited from counseling when they sincerely wanted to make an improvement. When people in counseling take it seriously, they tend to get a lot out of it."

Reassure the care receiver as necessary that a well-chosen mental health professional will not attack his or her religious beliefs. Effective counseling enhances an individual's spiritual life. Be sure to tell the care receiver that the mental health professionals you are recommending have been screened by the church's Stephen Leaders as people who are favorably disposed to people's faith and spiritual values.

Listen carefully to the care receiver's response. The feelings, thoughts, attitudes, and behaviors that the care receiver expresses are important, and they provide clues about what to say and do next. Watch the care receiver's body language as you listen to what he or she says. It might be appropriate to follow up in one or more of the following ways.

- Ask the care receiver to tell you more about his or her concerns about the referral, listen carefully as he or she does so, and then respond to those concerns.

- Reassure a care receiver who might interpret the suggestion for referral as rejection by you.

- Lovingly question a care receiver's belief that his or her situation will improve by itself.

Guide the care receiver through his or her decision making. Review the positives and negatives of the referral. Discuss any issues about which the care receiver has concerns, such as cost, time, confidentiality, or the continuation of the Stephen Ministry relationship. Be prepared to

> **To the Stephen Leader**
>
> Educating Stephen Ministers about typical costs of mental health care and assistance that is available to help cover costs may make a good topic for continuing education.

reflect feelings or ask clarifying questions that can help the care receiver sort out his or her feelings.

The choice of a mental health professional is the care receiver's to make. Offer the list of recommended mental health professionals, but be open to the possibility that he or she may have another professional in mind who does not appear on the list. Assist your care receiver in deciding what kinds of questions he or she should ask to ensure this professional is a good match. Help him or her have owner-ship of the final decision.

Also pray with the care receiver about the referral. Ask for God's guidance and help in the decision-making process.

Be both assertive and persistent. Don't take no for an answer. Build a fire under the care receiver, emphasizing the importance of this care, and gently and firmly insisting. If the potential for suicide, homicide, or abuse is present, the Stephen Minister must be very assertive and insist on getting help immediately. This may include calling 911 or making arrangements for family to take the care receiver to the emergency room of a hospital.

In situations that are not life threatening, assertively repeat the recommendation for referral several times during subsequent visits with the individual. Be patient and persis-tent. The urgency of the problem determines the frequency and emphasis with which you need to raise the issue. Keep the Supervision Group apprised of the progress or lack of it. See "Deal with the Care Receiver's Refusal, If Necessary" (on pages 110–114) for additional information.

For more guidance on assertiveness, use as a reference *Speaking the Truth in Love: How to Be an Assertive Christian* by Ruth N. Koch and Kenneth C. Haugk. The chapter titled "How to Make Requests" will be especially helpful. It includes guidelines such as these:

- Describe the situation as objectively as possible, based on what you have personally seen, heard, and experienced.

- Express your feelings about the situation, avoiding statements that would imply that the care receiver is responsible for making you feel that way.

- Specify the outcome you desire for this situation in a real-istic and positive way.

- Describe the possible consequences of the actions being considered.[1]

Remember, you are being assertive because you care.

7. Help the Care Receiver Make the Contact

Ideally the care receiver will make the first contact with the mental health professional. You may be with the care receiver when he or she calls the professional. In some circumstances, you may offer to accompany the care receiver to the first appointment, and perhaps even go in with the care receiver. Providing such support can help the care receiver overcome initial fears or reservations about working with a mental health professional.

While you should be as supportive as possible to the care receiver, don't overdo it. Encourage the care receiver to do as much as possible for him- or herself in making arrangements to meet with the mental health professional. The more responsibility he or she takes (e.g., placing the call, setting the appointment, driving to the office), the greater the chance of successful treatment. The motivation for care must ultimately come from the care receiver.

And yet . . . this is one of those instances when you must hold apparently contradictory realities in place. Yes, the motivation for care must come from the care receiver, but do your best to motivate your care receiver to see a mental health professional for a first visit. Then let the mental health professional do his or her job of motivating the person to continue treatment.

8. Deal with the Care Receiver's Refusal, If Necessary

A care receiver may resist the idea of referral to a mental health professional. If so, report that right away to the Supervision Coordinator. He or she or another Stephen Leader

---

1 Ruth N. Koch and Kenneth C. Haugk, *Speaking the Truth in Love: How to Be an Assertive Christian* (St. Louis: Stephen Ministries, 1992), pp. 116–118.

When and How to Use Mental Health Resources

may need to get involved or may have further recommendations to make. The Stephen Leader may present to the care receiver a more objective approach to the need for referral. When a care receiver hears about referral from more than one source, he or she is more likely to say yes. It is best to tell your care receiver in advance that you need to discuss the need for referral with a Stephen Leader. You can assure your care receiver that the Stephen Leader will keep this issue confidential.

There are several other helpful actions you can take.

Consult with Stephen Leaders and perhaps the pastoral staff about what to do next. The seriousness of a situation dictates the type and speed of action required if the care receiver refuses referral. For instance, in situations that are not potentially violent, abusive, or life threatening, it may be possible to encourage the care receiver over days or even weeks to consider referral. If, after a reasonable period of time, the care receiver does not agree to seek professional help, consult further with your Supervision Group or with Stephen Leaders or pastors who are already aware of the situation. Ask for their help in determining the next steps to take.

In situations that do involve the potential of abuse, homicide, suicide, or other significant dangers, consultation and action must be immediate. Safety supersedes confidentiality in such cases—neither you nor a Stephen Leader should keep a care receiver's plans for suicide secret. In a situation where professional care is imperative, a Stephen Leader or a pastor may be able to help convince the individual to seek professional care right away. If neither of those persons is available, it is essential and appropriate for you to consult with others who can help, including mental health professionals and emergency services through 911 or other access numbers.

Consider issues such as quality of ministry—i.e., wanting the best care possible for the care receiver—and legal liability when deciding how to handle an individual's refusal of a referral. It is best for you to share such decision making with your Stephen Leaders, pastors, mental health professionals, and sometimes attorneys.

Be cheerfully persistent. Be upbeat about what therapy could mean for a care receiver's well-being. Look for chances to point out, without pushing, the type of help a professional could offer. Don't be afraid to appropriately convey how the care receiver's needs require assistance that you are not trained to provide. For example, if a care receiver is describing his or her wide swings of emotion and asks, "Why do you think this happens? What's wrong with me?" you might say, "I really don't know. My cluelessness is a good signal that a professional counselor would be better equipped to provide the care you need right now."

Encourage the care receiver to give it a try. Just as some care receivers agree to give Stephen Ministry a trial period and are eventually glad they accepted a Stephen Minister, care receivers may also be willing to give professional mental health care a try and later be glad they did. This approach can help break the ice and get the relationship started.

Emphasize that seeking care from a mental health professional is a positive action. Point out that deciding to see a mental health professional means that the care receiver is perceptive enough to understand that some parts of his or her life need to change and is tenacious enough to go about finding a way to change them. Individuals who see mental health professionals often ask at some point, "Does this mean I'm really disturbed? Am I so different from 'normal' people?" One therapist responded to this question by saying, "Stand up and look out the window at those people out there. The fact that you're in here working on what's concerning you probably makes you healthier than many of those people. Many of them have significant life struggles but haven't made the choice to work on them."

Be clear about consequences. Avoid using scare tactics, but present the facts clearly so that the care receiver gets the message that you will be unable to continue as his or her Stephen Minister unless he or she follows up on the referral to the mental health professional. Gently but firmly let the care receiver know that you want the best care possible for him or her. Reassure the care receiver that you are not abandoning or giving up on him or her, but that he or she does need professional care. You might say: "I am determined to care for you in the way that is best for you. In fact, that is a good part of my job description as a Stephen Minister. That is why I know it would not be right for me to continue as your Stephen Minister unless a mental health professional says it would be beneficial for you."

Bring in others to help convince the care receiver, if necessary. As discussed in "Decide Who Will Talk with the Care Receiver" (pages 104–105), bringing in a Stephen Leader or a pastor may help. To introduce this idea, you might say: "If it's okay, I would like to have the pastor talk with you about this. I think the pastor could explain this more clearly."

Remember that in most cases it is the care receiver's decision whether or not to accept the referral. Except under very limited and serious circumstances, no one can make a care receiver get help. In most cases, the individual is responsible for obtaining assistance that would improve his or her ability to cope with and enjoy life.

If your repeated efforts to persuade a care receiver to accept professional help are unsuccessful, you need to consult with a Stephen Leader, pastor, or both to decide how much longer the Stephen Ministry relationship should continue. They, in turn, may consult with a mental health professional, if they haven't already, to help them decide what should happen next.

If referral to a mental health professional is obviously appropriate and just as obviously is not going to happen, someone in authority—a pastor, the Referrals Coordinator, or another Stephen Leader—needs to explain to the care receiver that it would be irresponsible to continue a Stephen Ministry relationship when another type of care is needed.

If the care receiver absolutely refuses to contact a mental health professional, you must end the caring relationship. At that point, someone needs to call a conference consisting of the Stephen Minister, the pastor, and the Referrals Coordinator to set a time to bring closure to the caring relationship. That meeting should emphasize that the care receiver's choice does not constitute a failure by you, the Stephen Minister. You will need continuing support from your Supervision Group and the Stephen Leaders to help you deal with your various feelings and frustrations.

9. Follow Up

Once the care receiver has agreed to contact a mental health professional, follow up with the person to see if the appointment has been made. If not, you can offer additional encouragement to the person to call the mental health professional.

the person responsible for seeing to the security of this documentation.

You or others can also follow up after the care receiver begins seeing the mental health professional. If the mental health professional has approved the continuance of the Stephen Ministry relationship, then your follow-up will take place in the context of your regular Stephen Ministry visits (see chapter 7). A Stephen Leader may also contact the care receiver after a time to see how the relationship with the mental health professional is progressing. If you and the care receiver have brought closure to the Stephen Ministry relationship, a member of the pastoral staff can contact the care receiver to see how he or she is doing.

10. Follow the Mental Health Professional's Directions about Whether Stephen Ministry Continues

After referring a care receiver to a mental health professional, you and your Stephen Leader have a critical responsibility: Follow the directions of the mental health professional involved regarding the Stephen Ministry relationship. For a number of reasons, a mental health professional may make one of a variety of recommendations concerning the Stephen Ministry relationship.

• Not to begin a Stephen Ministry relationship

• To discontinue a Stephen Ministry relationship already in progress

• To begin a Stephen Ministry relationship

• To continue a Stephen Ministry relationship

• To wait for a period of time before beginning or continuing a Stephen Ministry relationship

The next chapter provides information on why a mental health professional might make each of these recommendations. It also explains why it is so important for Stephen Ministers and Stephen Leaders to comply with the mental health professional's recommendations.

11. Continue to Provide the Congregation's Care

Whether you continue your Stephen Ministry to the care receiver, put it on hold, or bring the caring relationship to a close, the congregation has a continuing role in the care receiver's care, assuming the person so desires.

When a mental health professional asks that the Stephen Ministry relationship not continue, you must put it on hold or bring it to complete closure. This does not mean, however, that the church abandons the care receiver. The church continues to care in ways that congregations always care.

• Offering public and private worship to the care receiver

• Including the care receiver in Christian education classes, Bible study, small groups, and other opportunities to be with others in fellowship, community, and spiritual growth

• Giving the care receiver opportunities to serve others

• Praying for the care receiver (maintaining confidentiality as is appropriate)

• Providing the ministry of the pastor, other church staff, and lay leaders (such as elders or deacons) who have their own caregiving ministries

If the mental health professional says that the Stephen Ministry relationship should continue, the congregation also provides ongoing care as before through you, the Stephen Minister. You are available to the professional, with the care receiver's written permission, to share information about what goes on in the Stephen Ministry relationship. The professional might occasionally suggest ways that you can be a more helpful lay caregiver to the care receiver. Given permission by the care receiver, you may also contact the professional with any concerns.

Whether or not the care receiver continues to see you, the congregation can continue to support him or her in making a new beginning in his or her life.

• • •

All Christian caregivers, lay or professional, must be concerned with helping persons in need receive the most appropriate type of care for their situation. This requires being knowledgeable about the types of care available and the best way to connect persons with the care they need. Our calling to take care of the "least of these" (Matthew 25:40) demands no less.

7

A Stephen Minister and a Mental Health Professional Providing Concurrent Care

First Church has been involved in Stephen Ministry for 15 years. During that time more than 500 people have received distinctively Christian care from the congregation's Stephen Ministers. Most of these caring situations have been typical, with a Stephen Minister's care being adequate to help the care receiver through a difficult time. In a few instances, however, Stephen Ministers have worked with care receivers who were also seeing a mental health professional.

Last year, Sarah agreed to receive care from a Stephen Minister after her divorce. She was coping well until she learned she had cancer, and then her life seemed to fall apart. Helping Sarah deal with her reactions to both of these crises grew to be more than Amy, her Stephen Minister, was able to handle alone. Amy checked with her Supervision Group, which supported her through the process of referring Sarah to a mental health professional. The therapist believed that Sarah would still benefit from Amy's continued support and gave permission for the Stephen Ministry relationship to continue.

•••

. First Church's Referrals Coordinator was considering referring Tony to a Stephen Minister after the death of his wife. During the preparation interview with Tony, however, the Referrals Coordinator noted that Tony was very depressed. She first referred him to a mental health professional, who, after carefully evaluating Tony's situation, believed that simultaneous care from a Stephen Minister would help Tony's progress.

•••

Pastor Franklin talked to Allison after the death of her six-year-old son in a traffic accident. Allison told Pastor Franklin, who was a Stephen Leader, that she was already seeing a counselor, but would like to have someone with whom she could discuss faith issues more easily. Allison talked with her counselor, who contacted Pastor Franklin and gave his permission for Allison also to see a Stephen Minister.

•••

Lorenzo, a clinical social worker, was working with Mike, a new resident to the area. Mike had been experiencing serious anxiety as a result of difficulties adjusting to his new job and surroundings and was making good progress in therapy. Mike had just begun attending First Church regularly, and Lorenzo knew about their Stephen Ministry. Lorenzo believed that the additional support and connection with his new church would be helpful to Mike. After talking with Mike and receiving his written permission, Lorenzo called Pastor Franklin, who arranged for Mike to have a Stephen Minister in addition to his therapy.

•••

Mary had been seeing a pastoral counselor weekly to help her deal with her grief and depression as a result of her husband's death. Cassandra, her pastoral counselor, believed that Mary had progressed to the point where she could reduce the frequency of their visits and that Mary would benefit from the supportive care *of a Stephen Minister. Cassandra knew that First Church was a Stephen Ministry congregation and recommended that Mary, a member at First Church, call them. Soon First Church's Referrals Coordinator had arranged for a Stephen Minister to begin meeting weekly with Mary. Mary and Cassandra continued to meet monthly.*

• • •

Jim, a Stephen Minister, was meeting with his care receiver, Gary, with permission from Gary's counselor, Dr. Garcia. Dr. Garcia was helping Gary to deal with some difficult personal issues, which left Gary feeling very uncomfortable. When meeting with his Stephen Minister the day before he would meet with Dr. Garcia, Gary would share many strong feelings. Then, when he would see Dr. Garcia the next day, he didn't have much to talk about. This made it very difficult for Dr. Garcia to have much to work with. Over several sessions Dr. Garcia gently explained to Gary that it would be a good idea for his Stephen Ministry relationship to be brought to a close, at least for a while.

These examples, typical of Stephen Ministry caring relationships, illustrate some of the possibilities when a person receives care from a mental health professional and a Stephen Minister simultaneously and, in the last example, the occasional necessity of closing down a Stephen Ministry relationship. The purpose of this chapter is to help you and Stephen Leaders understand the kinds of situations when such simultaneous care is appropriate and to suggest some important steps to follow in setting up and carrying out such complementary caring relationships.

Differences in Care

Chapter 2 outlined the types of care Stephen Ministers can and cannot provide. It may be helpful here, however, to compare the various kinds of care offered by Stephen Ministers and mental health professionals. Although there is certainly overlap between the two, there are also significant differences.

Stephen Ministry is designed to support persons who for the most part have their basic coping skills intact, their thinking in order, and their emotions under control. They are usually able to meet the routine demands of everyday life. These care receivers have a reasonably accurate perspective about what is happening in their lives. Even without care from you, these persons would be likely to overcome their challenges, although probably not as quickly or as well. They need someone to walk alongside them and encourage them, to pray with them and bear their burdens with them. In short, they need someone to be Christ to them, and that someone is you. Your key purpose in a Stephen Ministry caregiving relationship, therefore, is to offer support through attentive active listening and a Christian caring presence.

In sharp contrast to lay caregivers, mental health professionals are equipped to work with people who are wrestling with issues that are challenging their basic ability to function. These clients' primary coping skills, if intact, are under great pressure and in danger of being compromised. They may be under such stress that they are not always thinking clearly and need someone to help them stay grounded in reality. Their emotions may be controlling their behavior and decisions in adverse ways. They may struggle to meet the minimal demands of daily living and fail as often as they succeed.

Like Stephen Ministers, mental health professionals may work with persons who are reasonably healthy, but they can challenge and equip such persons to explore their feelings and actions at deeper levels than they might otherwise be able or willing to do. Professional caregivers will often guide persons in examining their past for the roots of current difficulties. They can offer strategies for overcoming these challenges. Mental health professionals have the skills to help people change troublesome or destructive personality traits and behaviors.

When Might a Stephen Minister and a Mental Health Professional Care for the Same Person?

There are several situations in which a Stephen Minister and a mental health professional might care for the same person. Such a complementary relationship, however, can only take place with the express permission of the mental health professional.

Situations in Which Both a Stephen Minister and a Mental Health Professional Might Provide Care

• When a care receiver's life situation gets worse

• When a care receiver decompensates

• When a Stephen Minister discovers additional information about a care receiver

• At the time of initial referral to a mental health professional

• When a person already receiving professional care receives an offer of Stephen Ministry

• When a mental health professional requests Stephen Ministry for a client the mental health professional will continue to see

• When a mental health professional requests a Stephen Minister for a client as professional care is winding down

---

When a Care Receiver's Life Situation Gets Worse

Sometimes unexpected disasters strike in the life of a care receiver. A second or third crisis, layered one upon another, may push a care receiver over the edge. He or she may be unable to cope with the added burden, even with your help and encouragement. Professional help may be necessary, and certainly a referral to a mental health professional is in order. The mental health professional will then be the one to decide if the Stephen Ministry relationship should continue.

When a Care Receiver Decompensates

Decompensation is the six-dollar word mental health professionals use to refer to the deterioration of a person's ability to cope. The individual may have been doing fine, but matters get worse on the inside, in the way he or she perceives what's happening, and coping mechanisms crumble. A crisis that the care receiver could cope with, and for which the Stephen Minister was qualified to provide care, grows unmanageable for both of them. A mental health professional's intervention is necessary, possibly with a green light for the continued relationship with the Stephen Minister, possibly not.

When a Stephen Minister Discovers Additional Information about a Care Receiver

Sometimes potential care receivers are unwilling or unable to tell their whole story in their preparation interview with the Referrals Coordinator.

To the Stephen Leader

If you offer Stephen Ministry to a person and then learn that he or she is already receiving care from a mental health professional, your first step should be to ascertain the kind of professional care the individual is receiv-

They may be too embarrassed; they may think the Referrals Coordinator wouldn't believe them; they may believe the information is irrelevant; or they may be having difficulty accepting the reality of all that has happened to them. Whatever the reason for holding back pertinent facts, you may discover that you are not trained to provide care for all the concerns that your care receiver is actually facing. You will talk about this in your Supervision Group and with a Stephen Leader, and then with your care receiver to share your conviction that he or she primarily needs professional help and the mental health professional will decide whether the Stephen Ministry relationship should continue.

At the Time of Initial Referral to a Mental Health Professional

A member of the Stephen Leader Team interviews each person who expresses willingness to receive care from a Stephen Minister. As the Referrals Coordinator or another Stephen Leader speaks with the person, however, he or she may

ing, which could range from monthly medication checkups (with little in the way of therapeutic dialogue) to four-times-a-week psychoanalysis. A general principle: The more talk therapy that goes on, the less appropriate it is likely to be for a Stephen Minister to work with the person receiving care from a mental health professional.

The second step should be to explain to the church member why Stephen Ministry can only take place if the mental health professional agrees. The one in need of care should talk to the mental health professional he or she is seeing and ask if the professional would be willing to hear about Stephen Ministry from someone at church. (Of course, this preparation may have already taken place if this mental health professional is one of those your Stephen Leader Team has prescreened for referral purposes.)

Your purpose in speaking with the professional is not to pressure him or her into conclude that the person needs more care than a Stephen Minister can provide. In such a case, the Stephen Leader will refer the person to a mental health professional who will determine whether the care receiver could also benefit from the care of a Stephen Minister.

When a Person Already Receiving Professional Care Receives an Offer of Stephen Ministry

There may be instances in which congregation members experience crises, such as the death of a loved one or loss of a job, that would be ideally suited for Stephen Ministry. A pastor, another church staff member, or allowing the care receiver to meet with one of your Stephen Ministers. Your purpose should be to describe Stephen Ministry and to explain how care from a Stephen Minister might be helpful.

One caution in this situation: Do not harm the relationship between the care receiver and the mental health professional. If the professional decides against Stephen Ministry, be supportive of the professional's decision. Share the responsibility and express support for that decision when you tell the care receiver what the mental health professional has decided.

the Stephen Ministry Referrals Coordinator may offer the person a Stephen Minister, but find out that he or she is already meeting with a mental health professional. The Stephen Leader or church staff person will be very cautious so as not to interfere with the professional care the individual is already receiving. He or she may also explore the possibility of Stephen Ministry in addition to the professional's care.

When a Mental Health Professional Requests Stephen Ministry for a Client the Mental Health Professional Will Continue to See

Referrals by a mental health professional to a congregation's Stephen Ministry do not occur frequently, but they are happening with increasing frequency as more mental health professionals become aware of Stephen Ministry. This may be because the mental health professional sees the benefits of Christian care for his or her clients. For example, a counselor who is not a Christian may be working with a Christian client and may believe his or her client could benefit from the spiritual support offered by a Stephen Minister. A mental health professional may also request Stephen Ministry for a client because he or she believes the client will benefit from another set of listening ears and another caring relationship. A Stephen Minister can provide another layer of support for a hurting care receiver.

Either way, if the mental health professional knows that the client is a member of a Stephen Ministry congregation, after discussing the possibility with the client, he or she may contact the client's pastor or a Stephen Leader to discuss obtaining a Stephen Minister for the client.

When a Mental Health Professional Requests Stephen Ministry for a Client as Professional Care Is Winding Down

In most cases, an individual will make significant progress while under the care of the professional. For example, a person may have experienced a severe depression. Having responded well to therapy, which might include medication, he or she may no longer need the regular care of a mental health professional. The person could still benefit by further care of some sort, however. At this point, the mental health professional may refer the person to a congregation's Stephen Ministry while his or her relationship with the client winds down.

Stephen Ministry congregations are generally in a good position to provide such follow-up care. In professional circles, this type of follow-up is called "tertiary prevention." The purpose of tertiary prevention is to help persons leaving professional mental health care "to return their productive capacity as quickly as possible to its highest potential."[1] It is a crucial means of helping persons maintain mental and emotional health, preventing them from slipping back to their former level of inability to cope. Congregations, especially those with Stephen Ministers, are helpful partners in providing tertiary prevention since they can offer "a stable environment which can provide warmth, trust, and acceptance"[2] to a person moving out of professional care.

The Mental Health Professional Decides Whether or Not the Stephen Ministry Relationship Should Continue

To the Referrals Coordinator

If you are at the point of deciding about the appropriateness of a Stephen Ministry relationship, then clearly the mental health professional you decide to make a referral to is the one who decides on the acceptability of a concurrent relationship with a Stephen Minister.

The mental health professional treating the care receiver will decide whether or not the Stephen Ministry relationship should continue. A person's mental health care permeates all aspects of his or her life. A Stephen Leader Team, therefore, will seek the mental health professional's guidance and permission before assigning a Stephen Minister or allowing a Stephen Ministry relationship to continue.

---

1 G. Caplan, *Principles of Preventive Psychiatry* (New York: Basic Books, 1964), p. 113.

2 Kenneth C. Haugk, "Community Mental Health: The Role of the Pastor and Local Congregation," *Currents in Theology and Mission* 1 (1974), 60.

When the Mental Health Professional Is Familiar with Stephen Ministry

Mental health professionals make easier and better decisions about a possible concurrent Stephen Ministry relationship when they are familiar with Stephen Ministry. Once a congregation has compiled a list of mental health professionals to whom they might refer care receivers, the Stephen Leaders or pastors need to make sure that the mental health professionals on this list understand Stephen Ministry and its purpose.

When your Stephen Leader refers a care receiver to a mental health professional who already understands Stephen Ministry, the professional will be better able to make an informed judgment about whether that care receiver should also receive a Stephen Minister's care. If the answer is yes, the care receiver can ask the professional to provide a release form for the care receiver to sign that gives permission for the therapist to talk with someone from the congregation's Stephen Ministry. Then the mental health professional can provide guidance to you, the Stephen Minister, as necessary.

When the Mental Health Professional Is Not Familiar with Stephen Ministry

When someone who is already seeing a mental health professional is referred to Stephen Ministry, or when a person wants to see a professional other than one on the referral list, a Stephen Leader will need to explain Stephen Ministry to the mental health professional.

One way to do so is to use the "Sample Letter to a Mental Health Professional" in appendix C to prepare a letter to the therapist. This letter can help break the ice and clarify the goals of Stephen Ministry in relation to the care receiver. It lets the mental health professional know what to expect in terms of contact from the congregation's Stephen Ministry.

Another possibility is for the care receiver to give the therapist printed information about Stephen Ministry, such as some descriptive material that your congregation has available or even a copy of this book. After the mental health professional reviews the material, he or she might decide right then about whether a Stephen Ministry relationship should continue (or begin, if you are at the referral point in the process).

Still another possibility is for the care receiver to sign a release giving permission for the therapist to talk with someone from the congregation's Stephen Ministry. With this permission, someone from the Stephen Leader Team can talk with the mental health professional, explain how Stephen Ministry works, describe the Stephen Minister's role in relation to a care receiver, and answer any questions the mental health professional may have about Stephen Ministry. The goal is to provide the professional the information he or she needs to make a recommendation about the appropriateness of Stephen Ministry.

In instances where the care receiver is already receiving care from you as a Stephen Minister, you might go with the care receiver to an appointment with the mental health professional and further explain your role. (Of course, you would want your care receiver to discuss this with the mental health professional ahead of time.) Meeting you and hearing your description of Stephen Ministry may give the mental health professional enough information to make a good decision about whether or not you should continue to care for the care receiver.

One congregation printed a card similar to the one shown in figure 1 for care receivers to give to their mental health professionals.

(Name of Church)

(Street Address)

(City, State, ZIP)

(_____) _____
(Phone)

Stephen Ministers are laypersons trained to give Christian care to those in and around our church who are going through a period of crisis, e.g., bereavement or other loss, chronic illness, unemployment, and other life difficulties. This care consists of reflective listening and the use of Christian resources such as prayer and the Scriptures. It does not involve counseling, and Stephen Ministers are trained that they should listen and empathize, not tell people what to do.

Stephen Ministers receive 50 hours of initial training, which includes instruction in areas such as feelings, listening, assertiveness, maintaining boundaries, and confidentiality. They also receive regular continuing education.

Stephen Ministers normally meet with their care receivers for about an hour a week. They work under the direction of trained Stephen Leaders with the support of the pastor. They meet regularly with other Stephen Ministers and their leaders for peer supervision in which they support and encourage one another and hold one another accountable for their ministry.

Fig. 1. Card describing Stephen Ministers

A Decision about a Stephen Ministry Relationship

Once the mental health professional understands the differences between the care offered by a Stephen Minister and professional care, he or she will decide the appropriateness of a Stephen Ministry relationship for the client. The mental health professional will consider the nature of the difficulties the care receiver is experiencing and the nature of the professional care that the care receiver is receiving. Information from the care receiver, the Stephen Minister, Stephen Leaders, and the pastor may also be helpful.

Once the mental health professional has made a decision regarding the Stephen Ministry relationship, the care receiver and the Stephen Minister should abide by it in order for the treatment to be effective. You must remember that the overall goal is to provide the best care for the care receiver, and the mental health professional is best suited to make such a judgment.

Allowing Stephen Ministry to Continue Does Not Make the Stephen Minister a "Coprofessional"

The fact that the mental health professional gives his or her permission for the Stephen Ministry relationship to continue does not in any way imply that the Stephen Minister is now the mental health professional's assistant, or that the Stephen Minister is in any other way functioning as a professional caregiver. *Stephen Ministers never function as professional caregivers.* The mental health professional provides the professional counseling or psychotherapy. The Stephen Minister is a caring Christian friend who provides unconditional positive regard, reflective listening, prayer, and other distinctively Christian care.

If a Care Receiver Refuses to Tell a Mental Health Professional about His or Her Stephen Minister

If a care receiver refuses to inform his or her therapist about the Stephen Ministry relationship, even after repeated explanation and encouragement, the Stephen Ministry relationship will need to be brought to a close. To continue the relationship would falsely comfort the care receiver and be inconsistent with the nature of Stephen Ministry caring. An inappropriate caring relationship, with a Stephen Minister trying to care in a situation where he or she is not qualified, is even worse than no caring relationship at all. The congregation will continue to care for the person in informal ways so that the person will not be left with no care at all. Gently and firmly explain to the care receiver that his or her refusal to notify the mental health professional is the reason for the closure.

The Relationship between the Stephen Minister and the Mental Health Professional

When a mental health professional gives permission for a Stephen Ministry relationship to continue, the mental health professional and the Stephen Minister need to discuss how they will relate to the care receiver. Such a relationship requires cooperation between the professional caregiver and the lay caregiver.

Clarifying Roles

You, along with one or more of your Stephen Leaders, should probably meet or talk on the telephone with the mental health professional to discuss your role in the caregiving process. This will give you important information regarding the strengths and limitations of your care. This should be a brief conversation, or else someone may need to pay the mental health professional for his or her time.

Sharing Information

From the beginning of the relationship the care receiver, the mental health professional, and you must agree on the ground rules for sharing information about the care receiver and his or her treatment. The mental health professional will only proceed with this after acquiring a signed release from the care receiver. He or she may give you a copy for your records, or you can use the "Agreement to Receive Care" in appendix E of this book. With such a release, you can share any concerns or relevant information that comes out of your Stephen Ministry relationship with the mental health professional. The mental health professional, in turn, can provide you with necessary information or guidance on how to proceed.

Just because the care receiver has signed a release form doesn't mean that the professional will share all information that you or your congregation's Stephen Ministry requests. Trust the professional's judgment. A mental health professional is trained to know what to share, when to share it, and with whom. He or she will make the final decision about what is appropriate or pertinent to share.

If the Stephen Ministry Relationship Stops

Sometimes the different types of care offered by Stephen Ministers and mental health professionals do not complement, and in fact can interfere with, one another. This does not diminish the value of Stephen Ministry. If you end a Stephen Ministry relationship because a mental health professional decides you should do so, don't view it as a failure. It could indicate some very positive movement on the part of the care receiver, which you helped to facilitate, and it is the best path to the care receiver's future recovery and growth.

Prepare Care Receivers for the Possibility

Let care receivers who are also seeing a mental health professional know that the professional is the one who decides whether the Stephen Ministry relationship may continue. The mental health professional may recommend that the Stephen Ministry end, and if he or she does, the Stephen Minister will comply with his or her recommendation because it is in the best interests of the care receiver to do so. Discuss why this may occur and answer questions your care receiver has about this possibility the best you can. If you have prepared the care receiver for the possibility, the need to bring closure to your caring relationship at the mental health professional's request won't come as a surprise.

How Will You Find Out?

How might you find out that the mental health professional wants the Stephen Ministry relationship to end? In some cases the professional will relay this message to you through the care receiver. If this happens, confirm and discuss it with the mental health professional. In other instances, the mental health professional will speak to you or to your Stephen Leader first, with permission from the care receiver.

Who Will Tell the Care Receiver?

Who would tell the care receiver that the Stephen Ministry relationship needs to end? In all probability the mental health professional will carefully share this news with the care receiver. There may be circumstances in which the mental health professional would request that you inform the care receiver, but that would be less likely.

Dealing with Concerns about the Quality of Professional Care

If you are ministering to a care receiver who is receiving professional care, you or the care receiver may at some point have concerns about the type or quality of the professional care. It won't happen often, but it could happen. Tread very carefully in this area. By its nature therapy is likely to stir up emotions of discomfort—even turmoil—in a care receiver, and those changes can be good precursors to necessary growth.

A care receiver may say something such as, "That therapist doesn't know what she's doing! She needs help more than I do!" Most clients will get angry with their therapists at some point. This is quite natural; the client may be dealing with difficult and sensitive issues that have caused problems for a long time. If your care receiver is angry with the therapist, it doesn't necessarily mean the therapist is doing a bad job. It can mean that the therapist is doing a good job. The therapist's role is to provide what the client needs, not necessarily what the client wants.

In such situations, you must do what Stephen Ministers are trained to do best: listen without commenting, judging, or sympathizing. Certainly mention the care receiver's concerns in your Supervision Group. Be as supportive as possible in encouraging the care receiver's relationship with the professional caregiver. If necessary, help the care receiver be assertive with the therapist. Your care receiver has the right to ask questions about the type of care he or she is receiving, provided those questions are asked respectfully.

If the care receiver's relationship with the mental health professional continues to be a problem, especially if the care receiver is concerned about the quality of care he or she is receiving, you may consider a next step. Just as with physical health concerns, the care receiver might want to get a second opinion. If you suspect there are legitimate concerns about the treatment your care receiver is getting, turn immediately to your Stephen Leaders or your Supervision Group and ask for guidance.

While you need to be supportive of the mental health professional's work, you must also be alert to legitimate concerns about the professional's competence or ethics. The following warning signs can indicate a problem in the care receiver's relationship with the mental health professional.

Warning Signs

Be concerned about the quality of treatment if the professional does any of these unacceptable actions.

1. Exhibits unprofessional behavior such as shortening counseling sessions, repeatedly canceling appointments, or ignoring phone calls

2. Appears to be unhelpful to the care receiver after an extended period of time

3. Breaks confidentiality

4. Uses the relationship with the client for any sort of personal gain (beyond appropriate payment for services)

5. Asks personal favors of a care receiver

6. Establishes a personal relationship with the care receiver outside their therapeutic relationship while therapy is still going on

7. Becomes sexually involved with the care receiver

8. Involves him- or herself in any way with a client's finances

9. Pushes a care receiver into accepting treatment that seems unnecessary and may possibly be driven by the therapist's desire for financial gain

10. Encourages the care receiver to make major decisions, such as divorcing a spouse or leaving a job, without a convincing rationale

11. Encourages a care receiver to engage in behavior that goes against his or her personal beliefs or the ethical practices of your church or denomination

12. Attacks, challenges, or questions the care receiver's belief in or relationship with God (recognizing that sometimes a care receiver's religious beliefs can be disturbed and destructive and require questioning)

If these types of concerns do arise, you need to proceed extremely cautiously. Consult with your Supervision Group, a Stephen Leader, a pastor, another mental health professional, or all those. Someone from the church staff should be part of any consultation with another mental health professional. You do not and should not have to deal with such an issue alone.

With help from your Stephen Leaders, pastors, and other mental health professionals, you may identify and help address problems your care receiver is having with his or her mental health professional. It is important, however, to involve the care receiver as much as possible in resolving difficulties with a mental health professional. Where options for addressing an issue are available, present these to the care receiver and assist him or her in selecting the best option for his or her situation. If the pastor or someone from your congregation's Stephen Ministry were to immediately and totally take over in addressing problems with the professional caregiver, the care receiver might be left feeling weakened or inadequate. Obviously if the person feels incapable of dealing with such issues or is unable to take necessary action to protect him- or herself, someone needs to be an advocate on his or her behalf. Your primary concern needs to be the well-being of the care receiver.

There are likely to be fewer concerns about the quality of professional care if the care receiver goes to a mental health professional that your church has carefully screened and who has had a positive track record with previous clients from the church. You and others associated with your Stephen Ministry will certainly trust such a mental health professional more, and your trust will help the client trust his or her therapist also. Careful screening ahead of time is always preferred to having to deal with poor quality of care issues later on.

Comprehensive Care

Having a congregation's Stephen Ministry work together with mental health professionals is a wonderful opportunity to provide comprehensive care for the congregation's members. This is a concrete way to communicate Christian care for the whole human being. It demonstrates that the work of mental health professionals is not outside the bounds of the congregation's ministry, but is rather an extension of it. Close cooperation between a congregation and mental health professionals is important to ensure that all persons within a congregation receive the care they need. Such cooperation also allows each party involved to focus his or her energies on that which he or she is uniquely called and gifted to do.

The simplifier in all these seemingly complex variations of caregiving in the presence of mental health issues is this: What is good for the care receiver? What will provide the best quality care, the care that best helps the care receiver to be a whole, well-integrated, and growing child of God? With that as your focus, whether you are the Stephen Minister, the Stephen Leader, or the mental health professional, decisions about just which combination of caregiving would work best will clearly emerge.

Appendix A

Focus Question Set H:
Focus on a Possible
Mental Health Referral*

These questions appear as Focus Question Set H in the Stephen Ministry Training Manual *module "Supervision: A Key to Quality Christian Care." They are used during Small Group Peer Supervision, which takes place in twice-monthly meetings.*

1. What has prompted you to consider referring your care receiver to a mental health professional?

2. Have you noticed any of the following behaviors?

   a. Reduced ability to cope with life

   b. Symptoms of severe depression, such as uncontrollable crying, hopelessness, or inability to get out of bed

   c. Suicidal behaviors or the expression of suicidal thoughts

* For use only by your congregation's Stephen Ministry

d. Physical or sexual abuse to or by the care receiver

e. Extreme withdrawal

f. Hallucinations

g. Significant weight loss or gain

h. Abusing alcohol or other drugs or chemical dependency

3. Based on the "Referral Form" you received from the Referrals Coordinator, would you have expected your care receiver to be doing better by now?

4. Which type of mental health resource might be appropriate in this situation? (Refer, as necessary, to types and descriptions of mental health professionals in chapter 4 of *When and How to Use Mental Health Resources*.)

5. How do you think the care receiver will respond to your suggestion of a mental health referral?

6. What effect would a referral to a mental health resource have on your relationship with the care receiver?

7. What are some ways in which you could present the idea of a mental health referral positively?

8. If your care receiver refuses to seek help from a mental health professional, what will your next step be?

Appendix B

Confidential Stephen Ministry Mental Health Referral Record

Congregations and organizations enrolled in the Stephen Series may adapt and use this form. Before using this form, a Stephen Leader should consult with local legal counsel and with local mental health professional(s) as to the need and appropriateness of this form.

Date of referral _____

Care Receiver

Name _____

Address _____

_____

Home phone _____ Work phone _____

Reason(s) for Referral

Stephen Minister

Name _____

Address _____

_____

Home phone _____ Work phone _____

Person Recommending Mental Health Referral

Name _____

Address _____

_____

Home phone _____ Work phone _____

Relationship to care receiver _____

Comments Regarding Process of Obtaining Care Receiver's Agreement to Referral

Other Individuals Involved in Referral Process

Care Receiver Referred To

Name of agency or group _____

Name of mental health professional _____

Address _____

_____

Home phone _____ Fax _____

Comments about Referral

Form completed by _____

Follow-up to be monitored by _____

Dates for follow-up with care receiver _____

If Care Receiver Refused Referral, Indicate This Below and Briefly State Reasons

Note Any Chronology of Contact or Salient Facts and Observations Not Listed Above

Appendix C

Sample Letter to a Mental Health Professional

Congregations and organizations enrolled in the Stephen Series may adapt and use this letter. (See page 129 for information about when and how to use this letter.)

Dear *[name of mental health professional]*:

[Name of care receiver] is a *[member/participant/friend]* of our congregation under your care, who has given me *[his/her]* permission to write you. Our congregation has a lay caregiving program called Stephen Ministry. *[He/she]* desires to *[continue to]* receive care from a Stephen Minister, a trained lay caregiver functioning under the supervision of our professional *[and volunteer]* staff.

As noted above, Stephen Ministers are lay caregivers. They are not counselors, pastors, or therapists. Before they begin their caregiving ministry, they receive 50 hours of training in areas such as listening, dealing with feelings, assertiveness, and confidentiality. Subsequently they are involved in twice-monthly supervision and continuing education. They meet with their care receivers on a weekly basis to listen and be present with them during a difficult time.

We believe that someone who is receiving care from a mental health professional should have a Stephen Minister only with the permission of that professional caregiver. We want to be completely certain that we do all we can to promote [*name of care receiver*]'s spiritual, emotional, and psychological health and would not want [*him/her*] to have a Stephen Minister without your knowledge and approval.

[*Name of staff member*] of our staff will be contacting you soon to tell you more about Stephen Ministry and ask for your recommendation concerning whether [*name of care receiver*] should [*continue to*] see a Stephen Minister. We have asked [*name of care receiver*] to speak with you and sign any release necessary for you to discuss the advisability of [*his/her*] receiving this ministry. Our goal in calling would be to answer your questions about Stephen Ministry and get your recommendation, not to talk about any specifics of [*his/her*] case.

Thank you for your role in the life of [*name of care receiver*]. We want to support you in whatever way we can and provide effective care for [*him/her*].

Sincerely,

[*Name of Stephen Leader*]

Stephen Leader

P.S. *[optional]* The enclosed brochure describes Stephen Ministry more fully. I thought it would be helpful in your evaluation. *[Enclose a Stephen Ministry informational brochure, available from Stephen Ministries St. Louis.]*

Enc: Copy of *[name of care receiver]*'s "Agreement to Receive Care"

cc: *[Name of care receiver]*

Appendix D

Mental Health Resource
Information Form

The purpose of this appendix is to give you a tool for collecting information about mental health professionals to whom you might refer care receivers and guidelines for how to gather the information you need. Your thorough research ahead of time will give you confidence in recommending a mental health professional, even when you need to do so on short notice.

Adapt this form to fit your needs and then use it to name mental health resources, identify their services, and provide additional information. Then keep it in your congregation's Community Resources Handbook. *(Stephen Leaders can learn more about the* Community Resources Handbook *in "Using Mental Health Professionals and Other Community Resources" [T-11{1}] in the* Stephen Series Leader's Manual.) *Congregations and organizations enrolled in the Stephen Series have permission to adapt and use this form.*

Much of the information could come from the office staff (if any) of the mental health professional. Any information you expect from the professional him- or herself may be accessible in a 15-minute telephone conversation. For more time, be prepared to pay the mental health professional.

Pages 152–156 of appendix D contain the form itself. Following the form, pages 157–162 contain an explanation of some of the areas that the form covers.

Wherever you see a triangle (▲) on the form, you will find an explanation in the pages following the form.

Name of agency _____

_____

Name of mental health professional _____

_____

Contact person (if resource is an agency or group) _____

_____

Address _____

_____

Phone _____

Services Provided

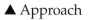 Approach

▲ Credentials of This Professional/Agency

▲ What types of service might this agency/professional be qualified to provide to a care receiver, or to Stephen Ministry (e.g., evaluation, general consultation, referral, or continuing education)?

▲ What fees does this professional/agency charge for services?

What type(s) of insurance coverage does this professional/agency qualify for?

▲ Describe the level of comfort this individual/agency would have in working with a Christian whose faith is important to him or her.

▲ How willing would this professional/agency be to work with a client who was also receiving Stephen Ministry?

Could there be a possible conflict of interest or tension between this professional/agency and Stephen Ministry? If so, describe.

Who (e.g., pastors, clients, colleagues) has endorsed this individual/agency? (Either list names here or attach letters of endorsement.)

Describe how a person would begin using this resource.

Other pertinent information

Researched by

Name _____

Phone _____ Date _____

▲ Approach

Questions about a mental health professional's approach may yield as much information about the professional as about the theory or methods that he or she uses. If the pastor or Stephen Leader who interviews the mental health professional is somewhat familiar with the field of mental health, it can be helpful to discuss the professional's approach. Even if the Stephen Leader or pastor is not familiar with the field of mental health, he or she can still use the responses of the mental health professional to determine whether or not to include the professional on the congregation's Stephen Ministry list of consultants. The mental health professional's willingness and ability to explain his or her work in understandable terms will reveal a great deal about this person.

While speaking with the professional, assess his or her manner: Does he or she speak in a patronizing manner? Is he or she direct and clear, avoiding jargon? Does the professional seem warm? Use the following questions to learn as much as you can about the mental health professional's approach to counseling.

- Will you explain to me, in lay terms, your approach to counseling or psychotherapy?

- Do you work with clients individually?

- Do you do family therapy?

- Do you do couples therapy?

- Do you do group therapy? If so, under what circumstances would you recommend group therapy instead of, or in addition to, individual therapy?

▲ Credentials

While credentials are not everything, they are definitely part of what you need to consider. A professional certified by an association is probably answerable to that association for maintaining certain standards of practice and ethics. He or she probably has had to meet criteria of experience and supervision. Likewise, if a professional is licensed by the state, he or she had to pass an examination that tests his or her knowledge of the field. Use the following to assess a mental health professional's experience and credentials. Most of these questions will be answered by the simple expedient of asking for a copy of the professional's vita plus any pertinent licensure information.

- Where did you receive your education?

- What degree(s) do you have?

- What has been your professional training?

- In what type(s) of continuing education opportunities have you participated recently?

- What certification(s) do you have?

- To what professional organizations do you belong?

- Have you been licensed by your state licensing board?

- What has been your work experience as a mental health professional?

- How long have you been practicing in this community?

- What are the sources for most of your referrals?

Based on the person's response to the questions above, you may also want to ask the following question.

- Do you receive supervision from one or more other mental health professionals? If so, who are they and what credentials do they have?

▲ Types of Service

As you build a referral list, look for mental health professionals who offer different types of service and different specialties so you can match care receivers' needs with professionals who specialize in those needs. Here are examples of questions to ask.

• What types of issues have you dealt with most in your practice?

• What area(s), if any, do you consider to be your specialty?

• Do you prefer dealing with particular types of problems? If so, which types?

• Are there any types of clients or issues you do not work with?

• What specific populations do you work with, and what services do you offer them?

• Have you consulted with churches and other groups before? In what subject areas?

▲ Fees and Payment Arrangements

Find out what financial obligations a care receiver who is referred to a mental health resource will face. Don't waste your time with the mental health professional asking these questions. These are examples of questions to ask the office manager, if there is one.

• What is your fee?

• Do third-party (insurance) payers accept your treatment and credentials as reimbursable? Which payers, for example?

• Are you a provider on any Health Maintenance Organization (HMO) or Preferred Provider Organization (PPO) plans? If so, which ones?

- What are your standard charges for telephone consultations with your clients?

- Do you have a sliding scale of fees depending on the person's ability to pay?

- What payment options do you offer?

- What would you charge our church for consultative services or for making a presentation at a continuing education session?

▲ Comfort with Christian Faith

Determine whether the mental health professional would be comfortable working with a Christian whose faith is important to him or her. A mental health professional who does not have the same religious orientation as the congregation or the care receiver should not be automatically ruled out as a caregiver. A mental health professional who is not a Christian can be the best choice if he or she is competent and respectful of the faith of others. Those who are actively hostile to religious belief or treat it as pathology are not good choices. Neither are those who are Christian but incompetent mental health professionals.

Following are ways to approach asking questions in this area and some examples of questions.

- Stephen Ministry works predominantly with Christians needing care. Our referrals to you, therefore, would likely be Christians. Would you be comfortable with clients who are religious in general and Christian in particular?

- If our referral to you needed to discuss his or her personal relationship with Jesus, how would you approach this clinically?

- Do you ever share your own spiritual or religious beliefs in a session?

• It is not critical to us that a mental health professional to whom we refer someone be a Christian. It is important to us, however, that when we refer someone, that individual receives good treatment that is not hostile to his or her beliefs and faith. I'd welcome hearing your thoughts on this either personally or professionally, or both.

▲ Working with a Client Who Is Also Receiving Stephen Ministry

Another obvious area of interest is how willing the mental health professional is to work with a care receiver who is also receiving Stephen Ministry. To find out, explain Stephen Ministry thoroughly. Share brochures and other publications your congregation uses to communicate about Stephen Ministry. You might also share a copy of this book. Say that you realize that it might not always work to have a Stephen Minister caring for a care receiver at the same time that that client is working with a mental health professional, and then get his or her ideas about how a Stephen Ministry relationship could affect treatment.

In many instances mental health professionals may explain that they would recommend suspension of a Stephen Ministry relationship while the professional relationship is in progress. There are well-grounded clinical reasons for doing this, so do not automatically exclude such a professional from the list of possible referral resources on this basis alone. Seek to understand his or her point of view, and include that as part of your assessment.

Here are some other questions that might be good to ask.

• Do any of your clients work with other caregivers while they are working with you?

• In general, what level of comfort might you have in working with a person who is also seeing a Stephen Minister?

- Under what conditions would you want or not want your client to see a Stephen Minister?

- Would you encourage a client to receive care from a Stephen Minister at the close of therapy with you if that seemed to you to be appropriate?

Appendix E

Agreement to Receive Care*

Congregations and organizations enrolled in the Stephen Series may adapt and use this form. (See page 133 for information about when and how to use this form.)

Since you will be receiving Stephen Ministry, it is good for you to understand the basic facts about Stephen Ministers and the care they provide.

What Does a Stephen Minister Do?

A Stephen Minister gives one-to-one, lay Christian care.

One-to-one: Stephen Ministers meet in person and privately with one care receiver of the same gender.

Lay: Stephen Ministers are trained and supervised lay volunteers, not professional counselors or therapists, pastors, or physicians.

* For use only by your congregation's Stephen Ministry

Christian: Stephen Ministers are Christians who care in the name of Christ. They are willing to talk about spiritual issues but won't force them.

Care: Stephen Ministers care by listening, supporting and encouraging, praying, being dependable and trustworthy, and maintaining confidentiality in their caregiving.

Confidentiality

Stephen Ministers keep personal information confidential. Therefore, you can feel free to share with your Stephen Minister without worrying that everyone else will know about it.

There are rare occasions when Stephen Ministers must share confidential information in order to save a life. Those occasions are suicide, homicide, or abuse.

Small Group Peer Supervision

Stephen Ministers meet twice a month in small groups to give and receive peer supervision, which is necessary to help them provide quality care and grow as caregivers. In supervision Stephen Ministers talk about their caring relationships and their own feelings about caregiving. They may share small amounts of information about their care receivers, but they never tell the care receiver's name and they do not share information that would reveal the care receiver's identity. Stephen Ministers may also receive individual supervision from a Stephen Leader or pastor, but the same rules apply.

Professional Consultation

On rare occasions a Stephen Minister, in consultation with a Stephen Leader or pastor, may decide that the best way to care for a care receiver is to consult with a mental health professional. In such cases confidentiality is strictly maintained.

Referral to a Professional

Some care receivers end up needing professional care. In such a case, a Stephen Minister or Stephen Leader will inform the care receiver and help him or her obtain the care he or she needs. That may mean that the caring relationship with the Stephen Minister will be interrupted or even have to end. When a care receiver needs professional care, the relationship with the Stephen Minister may only continue after the care receiver has met with the professional and the professional has given permission for the Stephen Ministry relationship to continue.

I, _____, understand the description of Stephen Ministry as explained in this agreement, and I desire to receive care from a Stephen Minister from *[name of congregation or organization]*. I further understand confidentiality in Stephen Ministry as explained in this agreement, and I give my permission to my Stephen Minister and to the Stephen Leaders and pastoral or professional staff of *[name of congregation or organization]* to give and receive supervision and to obtain consultation as described in this document.

Signed _____ Date_____

Other Resources from Stephen Ministries

To learn more about any of these resources or to order copies, visit www.stephenministries.org or call (314) 428-2600.

Don't Sing Songs to a Heavy Heart: How to Relate to Those Who Are Suffering

Pastors, lay caregivers, and suffering people alike have high praise for this warm and practical resource on what to say and do when people are hurting. Forged in the crucible of author Kenneth Haugk's own suffering, *Don't Sing Songs to a Heavy Heart* draws from his personal experience and extensive research with more than 4,000 others who have experienced suffering in their lives.

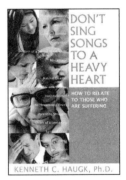

Don't Sing Songs to a Heavy Heart offers practical guidance and common-sense suggestions for how to care in ways that hurting people welcome—while avoiding the pitfalls that can add to their pain. This book combines sound psychology with solid biblical truths to touch caregivers' hearts and help them find the words and actions that will bring God's presence and care to hurting people.

For more information about *Don't Sing Songs to a Heavy Heart*, including excerpts, visit www.stephenministries.org/care.

Cancer—Now What?
Taking Action, Finding Hope,
and Navigating the Journey Ahead

Cancer—Now What? is a book to give to people with cancer and to their loved ones, helping them navigate the medical, emotional, relational, and spiritual challenges they may encounter.

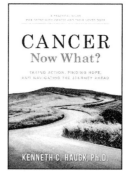

In writing the book, Kenneth Haugk drew on everything he learned as he walked alongside his wife, Joan, during her battle with cancer. He built on that foundation by conducting in-depth research with thousands of cancer survivors, loved ones of people with cancer, and medical professionals, incorporating their wisdom, experience, and expertise.

The result is a comprehensive, easy-to-read resource, written in a warm, conversational style and covering a wide range of topics relevant to people dealing with cancer.

Those who give the book include friends and relatives, pastors and congregations, oncologists and other physicians, cancer centers and hospitals, businesspeople and professionals of all kinds, and many others. For anyone wanting to support someone after a cancer diagnosis, giving a copy of *Cancer—Now What?* is a simple, powerful way to help.

A *Giver's Guide* is also available, which provides ideas for giving the book to those with cancer and their loved ones.

For more information about *Cancer—Now What?,* including excerpts and what people are saying about the book, visit www.CancerNowWhat.org.

Journeying through Grief

A set of four short books that individuals, congregations, and other organizations can share with grieving people at four crucial times during the first year after a loved one has died.

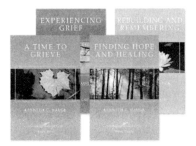

Book 1: *A Time to Grieve,* sent three weeks after the loss

Book 2: *Experiencing Grief,* sent three months after the loss

Book 3: *Finding Hope and Healing,* sent six months after the loss

Book 4: *Rebuilding and Remembering,* sent eleven months after the loss

Each book focuses on the feelings and issues the bereaved person is likely to be experiencing at that point, offering reassurance, encouragement, and hope through short, easy-to-read chapters. In *Journeying through Grief,* Kenneth Haugk shares from the heart, drawing on his personal and professional experience and from the insights of many others. The books provide a powerful way to reach out to a grieving person with four caring touches throughout the difficult first year.

Each set comes with four mailing envelopes and a tracking card that makes it easy to know when to send each book.

A separate *Giver's Guide* contains suggestions for using the books, as well as sample letters that can be personalized and adapted to send with the books.

For more information about *Journeying through Grief,* including excerpts, visit www.stephenministries.org/care.

Speaking the Truth in Love

This book invites the reader to live assertively, just as Jesus did. Building on a scriptural understanding of assertive living, it shows the reader how to develop healthy relationships with others—one to one, in small groups, in teams, and in congregations.

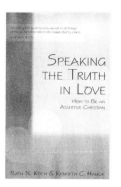

This deeply spiritual and practical book makes clear:

- what assertiveness is (and is not);
- the biblical foundation for assertiveness;
- how Jesus is our model for living assertively;
- how to be assertive in prayer and praise;
- how to make, refuse, and negotiate requests;
- how to express and receive compliments; and
- how to handle criticism, anger, and other tough relational issues.

Readers learn ways to relate to others with greater honesty, compassion, and respect—and experience the freedom and joy of Christian assertiveness.

For more information about *Speaking the Truth in Love,* including excerpts, or to order copies, visit www.stephenministries. org/assertive.

Christian Caregiving—a Way of Life

The definitive approach to distinctively Christian care

Christian Caregiving—a Way of Life explores the topic of distinctively Christian caring and relating. It offers practical skills for reaching out to others with Christ-like compassion, including how to: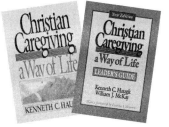

- listen actively and carefully;
- pray with another person;
- share from the Bible naturally and comfortably during a conversation; and
- speak words of comfort, encouragement, forgiveness, and hope.

Key themes in the book include:

- God's role as the *curegiver* and the Christian's role as the *caregiver;*
- the presence of God in the caring relationship;
- how to identify and respond to spiritual needs; and
- the connection between evangelism and caring.

The *Leader's Guide* provides discussion questions and other activities that turn the book into a course on Christian caregiving. Participants grow spiritually and build community while learning how to relate more effectively to family, friends, and others in their lives.

For more information about *Christian Caregiving—a Way of Life* and the *Leader's Guide,* including what people are saying about the course, visit www.stephenministries.org/caregiving.

Antagonists in the Church: How to Identify and Deal with Destructive Conflict

A ministry-saving resource for pastors and lay leaders

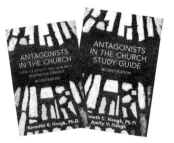

Antagonists are individuals who, on the basis of nonsubstantive evidence, go out of their way to make insatiable demands, usually attacking the person or performance of others. These attacks are selfish in nature, tearing down rather than building up, and are often directed against those in a leadership capacity. (From chapter 2, "What Is Church Antagonism?")

Pastors, church staff, governing boards, lay leaders, and others find the insights, principles, and practical methods in this book valuable for identifying and dealing with antagonists—as well as creating a congregation environment that prevents future attacks.

The *Study Guide* turns the book into a course to equip a group of church leaders to effectively deal with and prevent antagonistic attacks. It includes discussion questions for each chapter, which help course participants apply the strategies and concepts to their own unique situations.

For more information about *Antagonists in the Church,* including excerpts and a video featuring firsthand accounts by five people who learned how to deal with antagonists through this book, visit www.stephenministries.org/antagonists.

Discovering God's Vision for Your Life: You and Your Spiritual Gifts

Motivate and mobilize for meaningful ministry

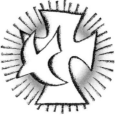

Discovering God's Vision for Your Life is a comprehensive set of resources that congregations can use to build a thriving spiritual gifts ministry.

The centerpiece of these resources is an eight-hour course that helps people discover, understand, and celebrate the gifts God has given to them. During the course, participants:

- learn the biblical foundation of spiritual gifts—how the Holy Spirit has equipped each of them uniquely for ministry;
- use the *Haugk Spiritual Gifts Inventory,* developed over six years by a team of social scientists and biblical scholars, to discover which spiritual gifts they have; and
- identify ways they can put their spiritual gifts into action—ways that get them excited to be involved in ministry.

As a result:

- people engage in ministries they're deeply passionate about;
- more and stronger ministry happens in congregations;
- more needs are met inside and outside the church; and
- people are drawn into God's vision—as individuals and as a community of faith.

For more information about *Discovering God's Vision for Your Life,* including what pastors and lay leaders are saying about this course, visit www.stephenministries.org/spiritualgifts.

The following four resources are Stephen Ministries Care Classics®—highly esteemed books on Christian caring and relating that Stephen Ministries has republished for the benefit of this and future generations.

The Promise of Hope: Coping When Life Caves In

by William M. Kinnaird

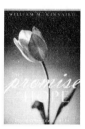

In this personal witness of faith and courage, Bill Kinnaird brings a message of hope to those who struggle and suffer. Amid the turmoil of daily life, he offers a place filled with reason, purpose, and the reassurance that God is always there.

Joy Comes with the Morning: The Positive Power of Christian Encouragement

by William M. Kinnaird

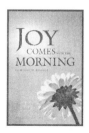

This book provides a wealth of personal insights and timeless ideas for Christian caregiving. Whether for daily meditations or study by a group, it helps readers experience God's love for and through God's people.

Yes, Lord
by Dona Hoffman

Poems, journal entries, and correspondence chart the journey of Dona Hoffman following her diagnosis of terminal cancer. Dona's courage, love, faith, and humor will charm and encourage both those who suffer and those who care for others.

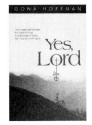

Caring Criticism: Building Bridges Instead of Walls
by William J. Diehm

This book meets a challenging topic head on: giving and receiving criticism. Combining Christian love and biblical principles, pastor and psychologist William Diehm shares practical, down-to-earth advice on how to offer criticism in ways that are helpful and non-threatening, how to receive criticism without taking offense or feeling crushed, and how to respond positively to criticism.

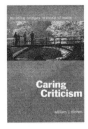

The Stephen Series System of Lay Caring Ministry

The Stephen Series (or Stephen Ministry) is a complete system for training and organizing laypeople for caring ministry in and around their congregations.

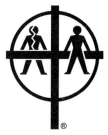

Stephen Ministry enables congregations to recruit, train, and support lay caregivers, called Stephen Ministers, who walk alongside a hurting person and offer high-quality, one-to-one, confidential Christian care. Stephen Ministers provide care and support to people experiencing grief, divorce, cancer, hospitalization, relocation, chronic or terminal illness, unemployment, loneliness, military mobilization, and countless other life crises or challenges.

More than 12,000 congregations and organizations representing over 170 denominations from across the United States, Canada, and 29 other countries have turned to the Stephen Series as a means of multiplying caring ministry.

Visit www.stephenministries.org to learn more about Stephen Ministry. If you have questions or would like to receive a packet of information about how to begin Stephen Ministry in your congregation, call us at (314) 428-2600.

Stephen Ministries St. Louis

Stephen Ministries is a not-for-profit Christian training and educational organization founded in 1975 and based in St. Louis, Missouri. Its mission is:

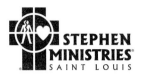

> To equip the saints for the work of ministry, for building up the body of Christ, until all of us come to the unity of the faith and of the knowledge of the Son of God, to maturity, to the measure of the full stature of Christ.
>
> Ephesians 4:12–13

Stephen Ministries' 40-person staff develops and delivers high-quality, Christ-centered training and resources to:

- help congregations and other organizations equip and organize people to do meaningful ministry; and

- help individuals grow spiritually, relate and care more effectively, and live out their faith in daily life.

Best known for the Stephen Series system of lay caring ministry, Stephen Ministries also offers resources in other areas, including grief, cancer, assertiveness, ministry mobilization, caring evangelism, church antagonism, spiritual formation, leadership, inactive member ministry, and spiritual gifts.

To learn more or to order resources, contact us at:

Stephen Ministries
2045 Innerbelt Business Center Drive
St. Louis, Missouri 63114-5765
(314) 428-2600
www.stephenministries.org